THIRD EDITION

POCKET GUIDE
FOR Lactation
Management

Karin Cadwell, PhD, RN, FAAN, IBCLC, ANLC
Healthy Children Project, Inc.
The Center for Breastfeeding
East Sandwich, Massachusetts

Cindy Turner-Maffei, MA, ALC, IBCLC
Healthy Children Project, Inc.
The Center for Breastfeeding
East Sandwich, Massachusetts

JONES & BARTLETT
L E A R N I N G

World Headquarters
Jones & Bartlett Learning
5 Wall Street
Burlington, MA 01803
978-443-5000
info@jblearning.com
www.jblearning.com

Jones & Bartlett Learning books and products are available through most
booksellers and online booksellers. To contact Jones & Bartlett Learning directly,
call 800-832-0034, fax 978-443-8000, or visit our website, www.jblearning.com.

Substantial discounts on bulk quantities of Jones & Bartlett Learning
publications are available to corporations, professional associations, and
other qualified organizations. For details and specific discount information,
contact the special sales department at Jones & Bartlett Learning via the
above contact information or send an email to specialsales@jblearning.com.

Production Credits
VP, Executive Publisher: David D. Cella
Executive Editor: Amanda Martin
Acquisitions Editor: Teresa Reilly
Editorial Assistant: Danielle Bessette
Production Editor: Vanessa Richards
Marketing Communications Manager: Katie Hennessy
Product Fulfillment Manager: Wendy Kilborn
Composition: S4Carlisle Publishing Services
Cover Design: Kristin E. Parker
Rights & Media Specialist: Wes DeShano
Media Development Editor: Troy Liston
Cover Image: © Dora Zett/Shutterstock
Printing and Binding: McNaughton & Gunn
Cover Printing: McNaughton & Gunn

Library of Congress Cataloging-in-Publication Data
Names: Cadwell, Karin, author. | Turner-Maffei, Cindy, author.
Title: Pocket guide for lactation management / Karin Cadwell, Cindy
   Turner-Maffei.
Description: Third edition. | Burlington, Massachusetts : Jones & Bartlett
   Learning, [2017] | Includes bibliographical references and index.
Identifiers: LCCN 2016012045 | ISBN 9781284111200 (spiral bound)
Subjects: | MESH: Breast Feeding | Lactation | Counseling | Handbooks
Classification: LCC RJ216 | NLM WS 39 | DDC 649/.33–dc23 LC record
available at http://lccn.loc.gov/2016012045

6048

Printed in the United States of America
20   10 9 8 7

DEDICATION

The authors would like to acknowledge the encouragement and support of our professional colleagues whose questions and experiences provided the parameters for this book. We are grateful to our students and the many mothers who have shared with us their breastfeeding questions, concerns, successes, and struggles. We are also grateful for the experiences we have had in our breastfeeding support groups and consults at the Healthy Children Project, Inc., The Center for Breastfeeding in East Sandwich, Massachusetts.

We wish to particularly thank our colleagues at the Center for Breastfeeding, especially our talented illustrator, Doreen, for the beautiful original art that is the basis of the new art illuminating this book; Vanessa Ford for the color consultation; Christine Rathbun Ernst for her careful review of the second edition; and Sheri Garner and Holly Hansen for their thorough review of the third edition. We are blessed with a wonderful "home team" staff whose support is invaluable.

We are very grateful to the editorial, copywriting, production, and rights and media teams at Jones & Bartlett Learning and S4Carlisle for their insightful, detail-oriented work on this edition.

Finally, this book is dedicated to you, the reader, with our very best wishes!

CONTENTS

Disclaimer   viii
How to Use This Book   ix

Section 1	Introduction	1
Section 2	How We Approach Lactation Counseling	7
Section 3	Normal Breastfeeding	13
Section 4	The Ten Steps to Successful Breastfeeding for Hospitals and Birth Centers	27
Section 5	Community Support for Breastfeeding	39
Section 6	Breast and Nipple Issues	43
Section 7	Breastfeeding Management Issues	77
Section 8	Baby Feeding Problems	95
Section 9	Can She Breastfeed?	161
Appendix A	The Healthy Children Eight-Level Breastfeeding Counseling Process	181
Appendix B	Feeding Observation Checklist	186
Appendix C	Breastfeeding Positions	190
Appendix D	Alternate Massage/Breast Compression	195
Appendix E	Protocol for Estimating Breastmilk Transfer	197

Appendix F **Protocol to Calculate Baby's Approximate Daily Needs** 199

Appendix G-1 **Table of Daily Breastmilk Volume Requirement Estimates (in Ounces)** 201

Appendix G-2 **Table of Daily Breastmilk Volume Requirement Estimates (in Grams and Milliliters)** 206

Appendix H-1 **Baby Weight Loss Table (LB-OZ)** 209

Appendix H-2 **Baby Weight Loss Table (Grams)** 214

Appendix I **Weight Gain Expectations and Infant Elimination Patterns** 217

Appendix J **Protocol for Building a Milk Supply/Relactation** 218

Appendix K **Protocol for Oversupply of Breastmilk** 223

Appendix L **Improving Milk Transfer** 226

Appendix M **Expression of Breastmilk** 230

Appendix N **Feeding Devices** 234

Appendix O **What to Do If an Infant or Child Is Mistakenly Fed Another Woman's Expressed Breastmilk** 235

Appendix P **Handling and Storing Breastmilk** 237

Appendix Q **Contraindications to Breastfeeding** 241

Appendix R **Breastfeeding Goals for the United States** 243

Appendix S	**Edinburgh Postnatal Depression Scale**	245
Appendix T	**The International Code of Marketing of Breast-milk Substitutes (WHO, 1981)**	249
Appendix U	**The Global Strategy for Infant and Young Child Feeding (WHO, 2003)**	251
Appendix V	**Innocenti Declaration on Infant and Young Child Feeding 2005 (WHO & UNICEF, 2005)**	253
Appendix W	**Glossary**	258
Appendix X	**Conversions**	277
Appendix Y	**Resources**	278
Appendix Z	**Pediatric Warning Signs**	287

References 289
Index 297

DISCLAIMER

There may be images in this book that feature models; these models do not necessarily endorse, represent, or participate in the activities represented in the images. Any screenshots in this product are for educational and instructive purposes only. Any individuals and scenarios featured in the case studies throughout this product may be real or fictitious, but are used for instructional purposes only.

The authors, editor, and publisher have made every effort to provide accurate information. However, they are not responsible for errors, omissions, or for any outcomes related to the use of the contents of this book and take no responsibility for the use of the products and procedures described. Treatments and side effects described in this book may not be applicable to all people; likewise, some people may require a dose or experience a side effect that is not described herein. Drugs and medical devices are discussed that may have limited availability controlled by the Food and Drug Administration (FDA) for use only in a research study or clinical trial. Research, clinical practice, and government regulations often change the accepted standard in this field. When consideration is being given to use any drug in the clinical setting, the healthcare provider or reader is responsible for determining the FDA status of the drug, reading the package insert, and reviewing prescribing information for the most up-to-date recommendations on dose, precautions and contraindications, and determining the appropriate usage for the product. This is especially important in the case of drugs that are new or seldom used.

HOW TO USE THIS BOOK

This handbook has arisen from our experience in helping new and experienced clinicians to hone their skills as breastfeeding problem solvers and counselors. We initially imagined this as a field guide to lactation care providers on the order of those available to naturalists and bird watchers. Sadly, our editors didn't think that the *Field Guide to Breastfeeding* sounded attractive as a title. . .

Nonetheless, we hope this book works as a field guide for you. It is not meant to be read from cover to cover, but rather, to be dipped into when you are working with an unfamiliar question or problem, or want to explore some other possible issues related to a familiar problem.

We use the term *lactation care provider* or *LCP* to describe those who are using this book. This term is inclusive of all who provide breastfeeding education, counseling, and support to child-bearing families, from those whose work focuses only on lactation to those who provide other types of services. Because scope of practice of lactation care providers ranges widely, please note that suggestions for treatment and referral of problems should be handled within the scope of practice of the individual reading this text.

Since lactation care providers come to this work from many different experiences, disciplines, and backgrounds, finding common terminology can be challenging. We have endeavored to express concepts as simply as possible. Terms that may be unfamiliar have been defined in the glossary, which is found in Appendix W.

The book is organized into 9 sections, followed by 28 appendices, a references section, and an index.

Section 1 introduces the role of breastfeeding in advancing public health, and explores the terminology used to define different intensities of breastfeeding.

Section 2 establishes our Healthy Children Project faculty approach to lactation care.

Section 3 identifies what normal, enjoyable breastfeeding looks and sounds like, and discusses the importance of following the baby's instinctive behaviors to establish a mutually enjoyable and rewarding feeding experience for the mother and the baby.

Section 4 briefly describes the Ten Steps to Successful Breastfeeding of the UNICEF/WHO Baby-Friendly Hospital Initiative, a set of practices that can optimize the establishment of healthy feeding relationships and mother–baby bonding during the maternity stay.

Section 5 reviews the crucial role of community support in building and sustaining the mother–baby feeding relationship beyond the maternity stay.

Section 6 addresses breast and nipple discomforts that breastfeeding women may experience, such as sore nipples and clogged ducts. The format used in this section follows for the remaining sections, including questions for the caregiver to ponder, other related symptoms or problems to look for, strategies for resolution, other concerns to consider, and some tidbits from our 70+ combined years of practice found under "In Our Opinion."

Section 7 uses the same approach to discuss issues women experience in managing breastfeeding such as timing, nutrition, and mother–baby separation during work or school.

Section 8 explores common breastfeeding problems from the baby's perspective, such as latch-on difficulties, breast refusal, and milk supply.

Section 9 focuses on other concerns that come up related to breastfeeding, such as maternal smoking, weaning, and illness in the mother.

Protocols for managing many breastfeeding challenges may be found in Appendices A through P. Other resources, including contraindications to breastfeeding, the Edinburgh Postnatal Depression Scale, and national and international policy documents focusing on breastfeeding, are found in the remaining appendices, Q through Z.

In addition to updating the evidence supporting many of the issues addressed in this text, we have made a few "tweaks" requested by readers—for example, adding many items to the glossary and converting the daily breastmilk volume requirement estimates appearing in Appendix G and weight loss percentages in Appendix H in grams as well as pounds and ounces. We have labeled these as Appendix G-1 and G-2, and H-1 and H-2.

We hope you find this pocket guide helpful in your work with breastfeeding families, and we welcome you to communicate with us about how the book works for you.

Thank you for all you do to get new families off to the best possible start!

Karin Cadwell and Cindy Turner-Maffei
Healthy Children Project, Inc.
The Center for Breastfeeding
327 Quaker Meeting House Road
East Sandwich, MA 02537 USA
info@centerforbreastfeeding.org

SECTION I
Introduction

BREASTFEEDING AND PUBLIC HEALTH

The need to improve breastfeeding behavior is a health priority expressed by the ministries of health in many nations as well as international authorities (Appendices U and V). In the United States, the Healthy People objectives (described in Appendix R) have included since their inception targets for breastfeeding for the year 1990.

Improving breastfeeding duration and exclusivity has been linked to favorable health outcomes in the mother and the nursling (Ip et al., 2007). According to a systematic review (Kramer & Kakuma, 2004), "available evidence demonstrates no apparent risks in recommending, as a general policy, exclusive (full) breastfeeding for the first 6 months of life in both developed and developing countries." Meeting the challenge of improving breastfeeding duration and exclusivity requires understanding the reasons women stop breastfeeding exclusively or give up breastfeeding earlier than intended.

EXCLUSIVE BREASTFEEDING, PREDOMINANT BREASTFEEDING, BREASTFEEDING, AND COMPLEMENTARY FEEDING

Exclusive Breastfeeding

Exclusive breastfeeding means that the baby is receiving solely mother's milk as its food source.

The World Health Organization (WHO) indicates that babies included in this category may also be receiving oral rehydration solution, vitamins and minerals, and/or other oral medications, but may not receive any other foods or fluids (2008). Public health goals, such as the WHO's Millennium Development Goals (Dodd, 2005), the U.S. Healthy People objectives (U.S. Department of Health and Human Services, 2011), and the policies of many health professional organizations, encourage exclusive breastfeeding for the first 6 months. After that, appropriate other family foods, especially those high in zinc and iron, should be added to the baby's diet while breastfeeding continues through the first year and beyond.

Researchers and experts from around the world have concluded that there are very few exceptions to the recommendation. These include:

- Babies diagnosed with galactosemia may not breastfeed or receive the mother's expressed milk. They must be fed a special formula. This is the only absolute infant contraindication to breastfeeding (American Academy of Pediatrics [AAP] Section on Breastfeeding, 2012).
- Babies diagnosed with phenylketonuria (PKU) may be partially breastfed, but also must receive a special formula. The amount of breastfeeding allowable will be determined by monitoring the infant's blood levels.
- Premature babies may require additional minerals, calories, and vitamins.
- Some professional organizations also suggest 400 international units (IUs) of vitamin D daily, starting soon after birth for all breastfed babies because they may not get enough outdoor time,

or they may live in parts of the world that do not offer enough sunlight exposure to manufacture vitamin D in their skin (AAP Section on Breastfeeding, 2012). In addition, they may have had sunscreen applied to their skin, which decreases their ability to make vitamin D. Concerns about future development of skin cancer have encouraged parents to decrease sunlight exposure of their children.

- Other medical or nutritional conditions may require additions to the diet of the breastfed baby.
- If the mother has a contraindicated medical condition (Appendix Q), is taking a contraindicated drug, or is undergoing certain radiation treatment, exclusive breastfeeding—or any breastfeeding—may require cessation, at least temporarily (see drug resources in Appendix Y).

Exclusive breastmilk feeding (EBMF) is a term used by The Joint Commission (2015) to describe the feeding of a baby with only human milk. However, the method of delivery of human milk may include delivery at the breast as well as via other supplementation methods (cup, syringe, at-breast supplementer, etc.). The ideal option for each baby is to receive the mother's own milk at the breast. If the mother's own milk is not available, donor milk from a Human Milk Banking Association of North America (HMBANA) member and/or a state-licensed milk bank would be the next best choice.

Predominant Breastfeeding

Predominant breastfeeding means that the baby is receiving the mother's milk as well as water, water-based drinks, ritual foods (such as teas), and oral rehydration solution, vitamins, minerals, and oral medications (WHO, 2008).

The predominantly breastfed baby is not receiving any other foods or drinks, including infant formula and other animal milks.

Breastfeeding

Breastfeeding means that the baby is receiving human milk as well as any other foods or fluids, including infant formula.

Complementary Feeding

Complementary feeding means that the child is between 6 and 23 months of age and is receiving both human milk and solid or semi-solid food. The introduction of appropriate foods, especially those rich in iron, zinc, and protein, is crucial after 6 months of age. Malnutrition starts at this age for many children, especially in resource-poor areas, which experience a high prevalence of malnutrition and stunted growth in children less than 5 years of age worldwide. The United Nations Children's Fund estimates that one-third of all children under 5 years of age living in low-income countries suffer from stunted growth (UNICEF, 2009).

According to the WHO (2003), complementary feedings should be:

- Timely, meaning that all infants should start receiving foods in addition to breastmilk from 6 months onwards.
- Adequate, meaning that the nutritional value of complementary foods should parallel at least that of breastmilk.
- Safely stored, prepared, and served.
- Appropriate in texture and given in sufficient quantity.

The WHO recommends that infants start receiving complementary foods at 6 months of age in addition to breastmilk, initially two to three times a day between 6 and 8 months, increasing to three to four times daily between 9 and 24 months, with additional nutritious snacks offered one to two times per day, as desired (Brown, Dewey, & Allen, 1998; Dewey, 2003).

BREASTFEEDING IS NATURAL, NOT INSTINCTIVE

In the past, the skills and techniques of breastfeeding were passed from one generation of women to another. Girls grew up watching their neighbors and female relatives breastfeed. Sadly, with the rise in the use of replacement milks from the late 1800s onward, breastfeeding knowledge and skills have become lost, muted, and distorted. Applying technology to the problem through strategies such as improving nipple graspability or distributing breast pumps seemed a plausible solution, but these strategies were shown by research to be ineffective in sustaining either breastfeeding initiation or duration.

Closer examination of the reasons why women stop breastfeeding before they wanted to points to the following:

- Concerns about milk quality/quantity.
- Feeding problems during the first week.
- Problems with their infant latching on or sucking.
- Lack of appropriate information and support (Ahluwalia, Morrow, & Hsia, 2005; Li, Fein, Chen, & Grummer-Strawn, 2008; Taveras et al., 2003).

In order to support breastfeeding as the cultural norm, all clinicians working with breastfeeding women and children should have access to education, coaching, and guidance about the management of breastfeeding. This book provides many resources and strategies to assist caregivers in helping breastfeeding families overcome common challenges.

SECTION 2

How We Approach Lactation Counseling

Together with our colleagues at Healthy Children Project's Center for Breastfeeding, we have developed a credo defining our approach, which we share below.

OUR APPROACH IS TO OBSERVE, EXPLORE, AND COACH[1]

We believe that:

- The mother, father, baby, and other family members know more about their situation and resources than we do.
- It is our job to observe, collect information, and explore the nature of presenting issues, and to coach families on the feeding and nurturing of their babies.
- As we seek to understand the nature of the presenting issues, other problems and concerns may be uncovered.
- In our conceptual framework (Appendix A), problems and symptoms are not the same thing. For example, pain with feeding is a symptom of a different problem—perhaps a poor latch or a tongue-tied baby. Through breastfeeding counseling, we seek to identify the true nature of the underlying problem(s), rather than to only remove the presenting symptoms.
- Once we have gathered enough information about the nature of the problem(s) at hand,

[1]Apologies to Linda J. Smith—we do not intend this to be an incursion on her well-deserved fame as "The Coach"!

we can formulate potential solutions, and propose them to the family.

- It is up to the family to then choose the solutions they are willing to implement and to carry them out.
- It is our responsibility to refer families for additional clinical or other evaluation as needed.
- It is our responsibility to ensure adequate follow-up for identified breastfeeding problems or to provide referrals for follow-up if it is not available at our workplace.

WHAT WE EXPECT TO SEE: HORSES, ZEBRAS, AND UNICORNS

It is our expectation that a mother who chooses to breastfeed will nurse her baby with joy and pleasure and also that her baby will thrive and grow on her milk. We also expect that she will breastfeed in an environment that supports her feeding choice. In other words, we expect to see breastfeeding as normal, common, and fulfilling for both mother and child.

When we see deviations from these expectations, we must be able to assess whether the deviations can be corrected by changing breastfeeding management practices or not. We think of these issues as horses, zebras, and unicorns. They all have similarities, and at first glance or from a distance—or without sufficient education or skill—we may not be able to tell the difference between a horse, a zebra, and a unicorn.

We think of horse issues as those that are fairly common and managed by changing breastfeeding practices. This book is filled with issues that are on the horse level. These are often-seen, everyday breastfeeding issues for which we have written "unique identifiers" in the text. We have offered suggestions on what else to think about if our techniques don't work. Perhaps the technique doesn't work because the problem presents at the horse level, but is actually a zebra- or a unicorn-level issue.

Example 1

A mother tells you that she has found a lump in her breast and has no fever or other systemic symptoms. There is a small area of redness observed near the lump that is slightly tender when touched. We offer her breastfeeding management strategies with the expectation that the lump will move down and disappear in 24 to 48 hours.

So, our expectation is that the lump is at the

horse level of the issue: plugged duct.

If, after 48 hours, the lump has not moved with frequent feedings, we move to the

zebra level: galactocele.

This requires closer scrutiny—imaging the lump and needle aspiration of its contents, for example. If milk is not aspirated, the lump may be at the

unicorn level: breast cancer.

Example 2

A mother has a reddened area of skin on her breast. She feels ill and may have an elevated fever. Our expectation is that the issue is at the

COUNSELING

horse level: mastitis.

If after treatment with anti-inflammatory drugs and antibiotics the area of her breast is still affected, the issue could be at the

> *zebra level*: recurrent mastitis with an underlying factor such as anemia.

Further investigation may reveal that the issue is at the

> *unicorn level*: inflammatory breast cancer.

Unfortunately, we have known mothers whose inflammatory breast cancer was undiagnosed for far too long because caregivers clung to the belief that breast inflammation in a nursing mother must be mastitis.

Example 3

What about a pus-filled area on the areola?

> *horse level of the issue*: infected hair follicle.

> *zebra level*: infected Montgomery gland.

unicorn level: herpes (can be fatal to newborns).

Sometimes, it is hard for caregivers to remember that breastfeeding is the normal, healthy way to feed babies. This is especially difficult if caregivers have seen a few zebra or unicorn issues recently. It takes a lot of effort to think on the horse level again. Or sometimes, caregivers are working in a high-risk situation and every breastfeeding issue seems to be a unicorn. This scenario can produce unnecessary stress for clinicians and the families they serve.

On the other hand, it is easy for caregivers to believe that breastfeeding is so healthy and that breastfeeding mothers are so well and that breastmilk is so good for babies, that they stay too long at the horse level instead of moving on to other, rarer possibilities (zebras and unicorns). Unfortunately, over the years we have had occasion to observe the sad consequences of this kind of thinking.

Thus we seek to understand what the normal breastfeeding experience is so that we can identify symptoms and situations that require deeper exploration. We explore the normal experience of breastfeeding in Section 3.

SECTION 3

Normal Breastfeeding

Babies love to nurse! Babies are capable! Typically, babies and mothers gain relaxation and enjoyment from breastfeeding. Pain and discomfort are not normal parts of breastfeeding, although they are, sadly, common experiences.

Normal breastfeeding begins at the time the baby is becoming hungry and the mother responds to the baby's visible hunger signals, also known as feeding cues. These signs begin during the active sleep state (identified by the presence of rapid eye movement [REM] in the baby). As the baby becomes hungrier and more awake, feeding cues are more obvious. The baby begins to bring his or her fist to the mouth; to seek food with the lips, tongue, and head; to smack the lips or extend the tongue; and so on. *Crying is a very late feeding signal.* By the time babies cry, they have usually become very disorganized and do not feed as well. Indeed, they may fret or sleep at the breast after only a few sucks.

GETTING STARTED AT BREASTFEEDING

- In the first hours and days postpartum, the mother and baby learn to breastfeed together, and move gradually from self-attached breastfeeding to collaborative breastfeeding.
- Each mother–baby pair moves in a unique pattern: one feeding may use self-attachment and the next collaborative. See **Figure 3-1** for more information.

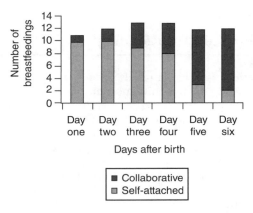

Figure 3-1 As mother and baby learn to breastfeed together, the self-attached feedings give way to those that are more collaborative.

- Mothers and babies move into a more collaborative style of latching and breastfeeding after the infant is able to locate the breast.
- During the first few days, the mother will become more and more comfortable with collaborative feeding as she and the baby learn together.

  In general:

- The infant's arms should not cross over his or her body, but rather should embrace the breast.
- In the early days, the infant's hands knead the breast during suckling. Hands should not be held away or anchored away from the breast by swaddling.
- The mother should not feel pain during the nursing, and after the feeding has ended, the nipple should not be misshapen, abraded, fissured, bruised, or blanched, all of which signal incorrect latch. If the mother experiences any pain, the infant should be gently removed and allowed to relatch.

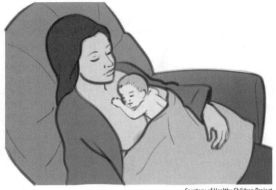

Courtesy of Healthy Children Project

Figure 3-2 Skin-to-skin holding.

Self-Attached Breastfeeding

- The healthy infant should be dried after birth and placed on the mother's chest for prolonged skin-to-skin holding, as in **Figure 3-2**, until the completion of the first feeding.
- The two are then covered with a warmed blanket.
- Maternal and newborn assessment, eye care, and other procedures are done with the baby on the mother's chest. (Note: Research shows that babies warm better in this skin-to-skin posture compared with electric "warmers" [Christensson et al., 1992].) The mother's breasts will increase and decrease temperature according to the infant's needs.
- Allow the newly born infant to find the breast and self-attach. This may take more than 2 hours if the mother has received labor analgesia. Mothers report that they enjoy having their baby skin to skin even if the baby does not self-attach and begin breastfeeding (Carfoot, Williamson, & Dickson, 2005).

NORMAL BREASTFEEDING

- Do not force the infant to the breast; doing so may stress the infant, decrease willingness to nurse at the next feeding, and cause the infant to place his or her tongue on the roof of the mouth (Widström & Thingström-Paulsson, 1993).

Widström et al. (2011) have identified nine distinct stages that newborns go through in their preparation for feeding. These stages include:

1. Birth cry
2. Relaxation
3. Awakening
4. Activity
5. Rest
6. Crawling/sliding
7. Familiarization
8. Suckling
9. Sleeping

Collaborative Breastfeeding

With collaborative breastfeeding, as the infant seeks the breast, the mother gently assists.

THE SEQUENCE OF SUCCESSFUL FEEDING

- Ideally, the newborn is held skin to skin or close to the mother so that feeding cues may be observed.
- When the baby demonstrates cues, the mother responds by bringing the baby to the breast without delay.
- The breast should fall at its normal angle:
    - The mother may support her breast so that its normal shape is not distorted.
    - **Figure 3-3** shows a rolled towel under the breast, which is a better choice than a hand if the mother's hand is observed to be distorting the nipple direction.

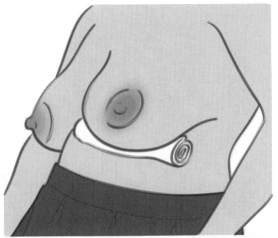

Courtesy of Healthy Children Project

Figure 3-3 Using a rolled towel under the breast can move the breast out and allow the nipple to be visible to the mother.

- ○ If the mother holds her breast during feeding (which is not necessary for many mothers), her hand should hold the breast still, and not obscure the place where the baby's lips will seal to the breast (**Figure 3-4**).
- • Collaborative breastfeeding may be initiated when the infant exhibits appropriate cues, including:
  - ○ Rooting—turning the head, especially with searching movements of the mouth and subtle body movements, as in **Figure 3-5**.
  - ○ Increasing alertness, especially REM under closed eyelids, as in **Figure 3-6**.
  - ○ Flexing of the legs and arms, and mouthing with little sucking motions, as in **Figure 3-7**.

NORMAL BREASTFEEDING

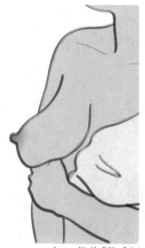

Courtesy of Healthy Children Project

Figure 3-4 How the mother supports the breast influences the direction of the nipple.

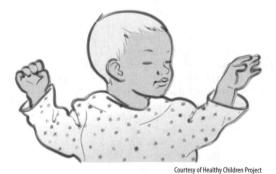

Courtesy of Healthy Children Project

Figure 3-5 Subtle body motions are a feeding cue.

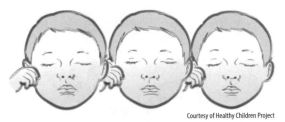

Courtesy of Healthy Children Project

Figure 3-6 Rapid eye movement (REM) is a feeding cue.

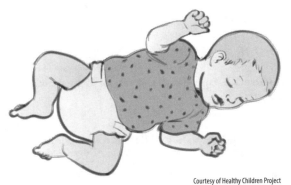

Courtesy of Healthy Children Project

Figure 3-7 Mouthing is a feeding cue. The baby may make little sucking motions.

- ○ Attempting to bring a hand to the mouth, as in **Figure 3-8**.
- ○ Sucking on a fist or finger.
- ○ Mouthing motions of the lips and tongue.
- • Crying is considered a late feeding cue because it does not usually begin in intact, full-term infants until more subtle cues have failed to elicit the mother's attention.

NORMAL BREASTFEEDING

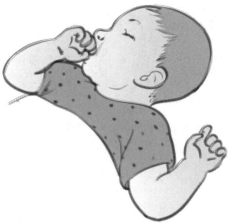

Courtesy of Healthy Children Project

Figure 3-8 Putting the hand near or in the mouth is a feeding cue.

- Less mature and more disorganized infants may pass quickly from the state of deep sleep (characterized by no REM) to crying.
- When using the collaborative breastfeeding strategy, the mother's body (especially her arms, hands, and torso) provides the frame and the support needed to keep the baby at her breast.
- The mother should find a comfortable posture and make her breast accessible to the baby.
- The infant should be allowed the freedom he or she needs to achieve pain-free suckling with maximal milk transfer:
  - The mother places the infant near the breast.
  - Her hand supports the infant's shoulder at the base of the neck, as in **Figure 3-9**.

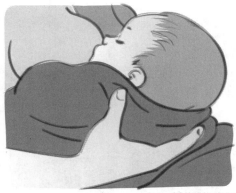

Courtesy of Healthy Children Project

Figure 3-9 It's important that there is no pressure on the back of the baby's head from the mother's hand.

○ There should be no pressure against the back of the infant's head from the mother's arm or hand or from a pillow; the baby must be able to tilt his or her head.

○ The infant's body is rotated toward the mother. This may be called "tummy to tummy," "chest at the breast," or "chest to chest."

○ The mother next moves the baby toward the breast, lining up the infant's nose at the nipple.

○ The mother's breast should not be moved to the baby; doing so may distort the ducts and impede the natural flow of milk.

○ Starting the feed with the infant's nose opposite the mother's nipple (**Figure 3-10**) assists the infant to orient to the breast via a well-developed sense of smell, and aligns the mouth at the breast when his or her head tilts back.

NORMAL BREASTFEEDING

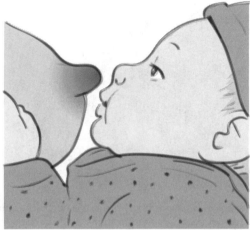

Courtesy of Healthy Children Project

Figure 3-10 Start with the baby's nose opposite the mother's nipple.

- ○ The mother moves the infant 1 to 3 inches away from the nipple.
- ○ As she moves the infant back toward the breast, he or she will gape, opening his or her mouth very wide as the head tilts back, as in **Figure 3-11**. If the infant fails to gape, the mother should repeat this maneuver.
- ○ Consider an additional session of skin-to-skin holding to improve the infant's motor state organization for the infant who fails to gape or nurse.
- ○ It is important for mothers not to push the nipple into the baby's mouth; doing so is unlikely to result in optimal positioning of the nipple or appropriate compression and release of the breast and nipple tissue during suckling.

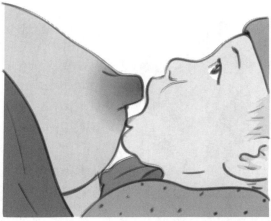

Courtesy of Healthy Children Project

Figure 3-11 The baby's head tilts back and the mouth gapes. The lower lip and chin reach the breast first.

○ The mother responds by moving the baby forward so that the tongue and lower lip seal first to the breast, followed by the upper lip. In this position, the nipple fills the open upper part of the baby's mouth, as seen in **Figure 3-12**.

○ The baby's mouth will appear off-center when compared with the areola. That is, the baby's lower lip will be against the breast much farther from the nipple than the upper lip. This is referred to as the asymmetric latch, as seen in **Figure 3-13**.

○ The baby seals to the breast and begins to suckle rapidly, perhaps eight or more sucks to one swallow at first, then shifts into a pattern of two sucks to one swallow or one suck to one swallow. This pattern changes during the

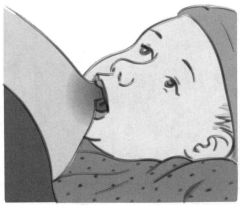

Courtesy of Healthy Children Project

Figure 3-12 The tongue takes up the lower half of the mouth. The nipple should be positioned in the top half of the mouth.

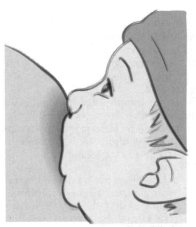

Courtesy of Healthy Children Project

Figure 3-13 The baby is positioned asymmetrically at the breast.

course of the feed, with the periods of 2:1 or 1:1 reflecting times of greater milk transfer. These periods are interspersed with more rapid sucking sequences and occasional rest periods.

○ After the colostral stage, the baby can transfer several ounces of milk in very few minutes when appropriately latched and hungry. There is no right length of feed to ensure adequate milk transfer. However, babies with consistently short (< 5 minutes) or long (> 20 minutes) feeds should be assessed to ensure adequate milk transfer.

• Breastfeeding sessions are best ended by the infant. When the feeding ends, the infant is relaxed, as in **Figure 3-14**, hands are open

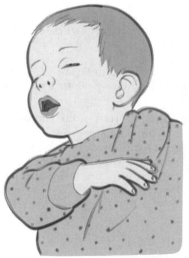

Courtesy of Healthy Children Project

Figure 3-14 When the baby has had enough milk, the hands and body are relaxed.

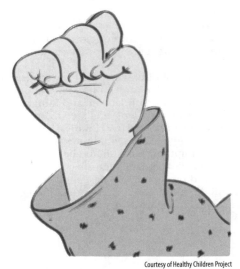

Courtesy of Healthy Children Project

Figure 3-15 Hungry babies have clenched fists.

(i.e., not clenched as in **Figure 3-15**), the arms are floppy, the brow is smooth, and the toes are curled.

The ultimate proof of the success of breast-feeding is a baby who is growing well, producing numerous wet and dirty diapers, and enjoying a close relationship with the mother and her partner. See Appendix I for more specifics about what is expected.

SECTION 4

The Ten Steps to Successful Breastfeeding for Hospitals and Birth Centers

The Ten Steps to Successful Breastfeeding for Hospitals and Birth Centers are the basis for the UNICEF/WHO Baby-Friendly Hospital Initiative (BFHI). The steps for the United States are as follows:

1. Have a written breastfeeding policy that is routinely communicated to all healthcare staff.
2. Train all healthcare staff in the skills necessary to implement this policy.
3. Inform all pregnant women about the benefits and management of breastfeeding.
4. Help mothers initiate breastfeeding within one hour of birth.[1]
5. Show mothers how to breastfeed and how to maintain lactation, even if they are separated from their infants.
6. Give infants no food or drink other than breast-milk, unless medically indicated.
7. Practice rooming in—allow mothers and infants to remain together 24 hours a day.
8. Encourage breastfeeding on demand.
9. Give no pacifiers or artificial nipples to breastfeeding infants.

---

[1] This step is now interpreted as: Place babies in skin-to-skin contact with their mothers immediately following birth for at least an hour and encourage mothers to recognize when their babies are ready to breastfeed, offering help if needed. (Baby-Friendly USA, 2010)

10. Foster the establishment of breastfeeding support groups, and refer mothers to them on discharge from the hospital or birth center. (Baby-Friendly USA, n.d.)

The BFHI encourages hospitals and birthing centers to develop policies and implement practices that support mothers in their choice to breastfeed. National authorities recognize hospitals and birthing centers when they have fully implemented the Ten Steps to Successful Breastfeeding. Baby-Friendly USA, Inc., is the designated national authority in the United States. Through this organization, maternity facilities signify their commitment to implementing the Ten Steps by following the 4-D Pathway (Discovery, Development, Dissemination, and Designation).

Being designated as a Baby-Friendly facility requires an onsite survey by a Baby-Friendly assessment team after the hospital or birthing center and the national authority indicate readiness for assessment.

The following is a brief synopsis of the expectations of each of the Ten Steps. For more information, consult the WHO/UNICEF International (2009) and Baby-Friendly USA (2010) guidelines.

STEP 1
Have a written breastfeeding policy that is routinely communicated to all healthcare staff.

Purpose
Ensure that policy exists that promotes breastfeeding and delineates standards of care for breastfeeding mothers and babies.

Criteria

The facility will have a detailed breastfeeding policy that is inclusive of the Ten Steps to Successful Breastfeeding, and will ensure that it is routinely communicated to all healthcare staff.

Healthcare facility staff member responsibilities include:
- Being oriented to the facility's breastfeeding policy.
- Knowing where the breastfeeding policy is kept and how to access the policy.
- Knowing what the breastfeeding policy covers, and what his or her responsibilities are under the policy.
- Being able to competently perform any procedures and practices identified in the breastfeeding policy as part of his or her job description.

STEP 2

Train all healthcare staff in skills necessary to implement this policy.

Purpose

Ensure that all staff have the knowledge and skill necessary to provide quality breastfeeding care.

Criteria

All staff with primary responsibility for the care of breastfeeding mothers and babies will have a minimum of 20 hours of training, including 3 or more hours of competency verification. Training for other staff members may be tailored to their job description and degree of exposure to breastfeeding.

Healthcare facility staff member responsibilities include:
- Participating in learning activities that address the requirements of the BFHI.

- Documenting learning in the facility's designated record.
- Demonstrating competency in selected procedures.
- Documenting competency in the facility's designated record.

STEP 3

Inform all pregnant women about the benefits and management of breastfeeding.

Purpose

Ensure the integration of messages about breastfeeding in all prenatal education interchanges.

Criteria

All women delivering in the facility will have received consistent, positive messages about breastfeeding through prenatal education. Topics to be covered include the benefits of breastfeeding, the importance of exclusive breastfeeding, and the basics of breastfeeding management (such as skin-to-skin contact, rooming-in, feeding on cue) as well as the possible effect of analgesia/anesthesia on infant behavior and the availability of nonpharmacologic pain relief. Mothers-to-be should know that their companion of choice is welcome during labor and birth. All prenatal educational media should be free of messages that promote artificial feeding.

Prenatal/antenatal staff members should demonstrate competency in:

- Educating and counseling pregnant women regarding the topics identified in the preceding criteria section.

STEP 4

Help all mothers initiate breastfeeding within 1 hour of birth. (This step is now interpreted as follows: Place babies in skin-to-skin contact with their mothers immediately following birth for at least an hour, and encourage mothers to recognize when their babies are ready to breast-feed, offering help if needed [Baby-Friendly USA, Inc., 2010].)

Purpose

Ensure the early initiation of skin-to-skin contact for all babies (whether or not there is an intention to breastfeed), and the early initiation of breastfeeding for those who intend to.

Criteria

All healthy, full-term babies should be placed in their mother's arms, skin to skin, immediately after birth and held there continuously and uninterrupted until the completion of the first feeding. Staff should offer assistance during this period to help the parents learn and respond to the infant's nine stages. In the event of cesarean birth, babies should be placed, skin to skin, in the mother's arms as soon as the mother is able to respond to her baby.

Labor and delivery staff members should demonstrate competency in:

- Encouraging and protecting continuous, uninterrupted skin-to-skin contact for all healthy infants in the hour after birth.
- Encouraging and protecting placement of healthy babies skin to skin after cesarean birth, as soon as the mother is safely able to respond to her baby.

- Educating and coaching parents regarding observing and responding to the feeding cues of healthy infants.

STEP 5
Show mothers how to breastfeed and how to maintain lactation even if they should be separated from their infants.

Purpose
Ensure ongoing breastfeeding assessment, evaluation, and support during the stay.

Criteria
All mothers should receive additional assistance with breastfeeding in the first 6 hours after birth and throughout the maternity stay. Staff should routinely assess mother–baby comfort and effectiveness of feeding and suggest changes as needed. Education should be offered regarding feeding in response to infant cues and methods of expressing breastmilk. Mothers of preterm or ill babies should be educated about collecting their milk via hand (manual) expression and/or pumping.

Postpartum staff members should demonstrate competency in:
- Assisting mothers to breastfeed within the first hours after birth.
- Performing routine assessment of the comfort of the mother and baby and the effectiveness of breastfeeding.
- Identifying and educating mothers about changes in breastfeeding technique as needed.
- Educating families about feeding in response to infant cues.

- Educating mothers about methods of expressing breastmilk, including hand expression.
- Educating mothers of preterm or ill babies about collecting and storing their milk according to the requirements of the special care nursery.
- Educating formula-feeding parents about safely mixing, storing, and feeding infant formula.

STEP 6

Give newborn infants no food or drink other than breastmilk, unless medically indicated.

Purpose

Ensure that healthy breastfeeding babies are not routinely supplemented with any food or drink other than human milk (unless medical indications exist for supplementation), and protect parents from formula marketing.

Criteria

All breastfed infants will be exclusively breastfed except when (1) acceptable medical indications exist for supplementation or (2) parents request supplementation after receiving education regarding the possible consequences of supplementation that is not clinically indicated. Parents of breastfed infants will receive no free samples, items bearing formula company names or logos, coupons for formula, and so on.

Postpartum staff member responsibilities include:

- Correctly defining "exclusive" breastfeeding.
- Identifying acceptable clinical indications for supplementation.
- Demonstrating competency in educating/counseling parents about the possible consequences of nonindicated supplementation.

THE TEN STEPS

STEP 7

Practice rooming-in to allow mothers and infants to remain together 24 hours a day.

Purpose

Ensure that healthy mothers and babies have ample opportunities for skin-to-skin contact, and ensure that mothers achieve early learning of the baby's feeding cues.

Criteria

Rooming-in should be practiced throughout the facility. There should be no routine delays between birth and the initiation of continuous mother–baby contact. Mothers who ask to have their babies taken to the nursery should receive information about the rationale for rooming-in. Healthy mothers and babies should not be routinely separated during their stay, with the exception of up to 1 hour daily for any clinically necessary procedures.

Postpartum staff member responsibilities include:

- Ensuring competency in educating/counseling mothers regarding the hospital/birth facility's rooming-in policy.
- Working to prevent routine delays between birth and the initiation of continuous mother–baby contact.
- Ensuring competency in educating/counseling mothers who request separation from their babies about the rationale for rooming-in, with the exception of up to 1 hour daily for any medically necessary procedures.

STEP 8

Encourage breastfeeding on demand.

Purpose

Ensure that mothers are encouraged to feed their babies in response to the baby's signs of feeding readiness.

Criteria

All mothers should be educated about the baby's ability to indicate feeding readiness and self-regulate feedings when given unlimited learning opportunities. Staff should assist families in the process of learning about feeding cues and responding to them. Mothers should not be told to feed on any particular schedule or interval, but rather to expect a minimum of 10 to 12 feedings in 24 hours with no particular pattern of frequency.

Postpartum staff members should demonstrate competency in:
- Educating/counseling families regarding the baby's ability to indicate feeding readiness and self-regulate feedings when given unlimited learning opportunities.
- Educating/counseling families in the process of responding to feeding cues.
- Educating/counseling mothers to expect a minimum of 10 to 12 feedings in 24 hours with no particular pattern of frequency.

STEP 9
Give no artificial teat or pacifiers.

Purpose

Ensure that breastfed babies are not deterred from learning how to suckle at the breast and thereby from maximizing mothers' milk supply.

THE TEN STEPS

Criteria

Healthcare staff should not offer healthy, breastfed babies pacifiers or artificial nipples. (There may be a role for pacifier use in the preterm or ill baby who is not able to suckle at the breast, or for the brief use of pacifiers during painful procedures during which holding or nursing the baby is not an option.) When breastfed infants require supplementation, efforts should be made to limit the supplementation device to a cup, tube, or syringe to avoid introducing artificial nipple shapes.

Postpartum staff members should demonstrate competency in:

- Educating/counseling families regarding the appropriate use of pacifiers and bottle nipples for the breastfed baby.
- Helping parents to provide supplements by cup, tube, or syringe as specified by hospital/birth center policy, when the need for supplementation is clinically indicated.

STEP 10

Foster the establishment of breastfeeding support groups, and refer mothers to them on discharge from the hospital or clinic.

Purpose

Ensure that mothers are linked to ongoing breastfeeding support resources.

Criteria

Facilities should assess the available community breastfeeding support resources and foster the development of breastfeeding support networks. All mothers should receive referral to appropriate community resources prior to their discharge. Staff should develop individual care plans for the follow-up of mothers and babies who have identified breastfeeding risk factors.

Postpartum staff members should demonstrate competency in:
- Identifying breastfeeding risk factors and developing individual care plans for the follow-up of mothers and babies with identified breastfeeding risks.
- Identifying available community breastfeeding support resources, and referring mothers appropriately prior to discharge.

COMPLIANCE WITH THE INTERNATIONAL CODE OF MARKETING OF BREAST-MILK SUBSTITUTES

The International Code of Marketing of Breast-Milk Substitutes was adopted by the World Health Assembly in 1981 as a piece of model legislation intended to be implemented internationally, but is not currently in force in the United States (see Appendix T for more information). This additional step requires that the facility purchase infant formula and feeding devices in the same manner used to procure other food and supplies, and that facility staff interact with childbearing families and vendors of items covered by the code in a specific fashion to promote, protect, and support breastfeeding in the face of competing commercial agendas.

Administrative staff responsibilities include:
- Ensuring that manufacturers and distributors of products that may be used as breastmilk substitutes as well as feeding devices for such have

THE TEN STEPS

no direct contact with the pregnant women and families served by the facility.

- Ensuring that the interaction of representatives of companies covered by the code and facility administration and staff are in compliance with the facility's vendor policy.
- Verifying that all infant formula and related feeding items used to feed infants and distributed to childbearing families throughout the facility are purchased at a fair market price.
- Ensuring that the hospital/birth center contains no items bearing formula company names or logos, and ensuring that breastfeeding parents are not given formula discharge bags, coupons for formula, or formula to take home from the hospital without a medical indication.

Maternity staff responsibilities include:

- Verifying that all prenatal educational information provided to new families is free of messages that promote artificial feeding.

SECTION 5

Community Support for Breastfeeding

Prenatal/antenatal interactions should:
- Include both professional and lay encouragement to consider breastfeeding.
- Elicit and address the individual reasons the mother and her supporters are attracted to breastfeeding.
- Elicit and address the individual concerns of the mother and her supporters.
- Provide opportunities for the mother to observe and ask questions of breastfeeding mothers with young babies.
- Provide information about facilitating postpartum breastfeeding management strategies, including:
  - Skin-to-skin holding.
  - Self-attached and collaborative feeding techniques.
  - Recognizing feeding cues.
  - Feeding on cue.
  - Feeding frequency.
  - Rooming-in.
  - Use of supplements.
  - Use of pacifiers.
- Provide opportunities for the mother to visualize how breastfeeding will fit into her life.
- Provide opportunities for the mother to establish friendship ties with other pregnant women with close due dates.
- Provide information about postpartum community breastfeeding support.

Factors that discourage women from breastfeeding:

- Coupons, bags, and other free "gifts" from manufacturers of breastmilk substitutes.
- Breastmilk substitutes advertised in magazines and on television as the cultural norm while breastfeeding is discouraged in public.
- Family members and peers who may discourage women from breastfeeding.
- Fear of pain and embarrassment.
- Fears about the adequacy of milk supply.
- Fears about inadequacy of breast size or appearance.

Factors that affect the duration of breastfeeding:

- Scheduled, delayed, or "timed" feedings.
- Inadequate number of feedings.
- Inadequate transfer of breastmilk to the baby.
- Inverted nipple that does not evert during suckling.
- Mother's fear that she does not have enough milk. This is also a common reason for the introduction of breastmilk substitutes and weaning foods before the recommended age of around 6 months.
- Breast surgery that has damaged lactiferous ducts and/or breast/nipple innervation or circulation.
- Infants with an inadequate suck, such as premies or infants with facial or other anomalies that reduce the infant's ability to feed effectively.

Postpartum community support for breastfeeding mothers should:

- Include both professional and lay breastfeeding education and support.
- Be communicated to pregnant women as well as to new mothers prior to hospital/birth center discharge.

- Include lay as well as professional support, education, and follow-up.
- Include assessment of an entire breastfeed, including prefeeding behaviors.
- Include prompt referral to primary healthcare provider, if needed.

SECTION 6

Breast and Nipple Issues

CONCERN: HISTORY OF BREAST SURGERY/INJURY

Descriptor: Breast Augmentation

Women who have had breast augmentation have a greater chance of lactation insufficiency than women who have not. The periareolar incision is most significantly associated with lactation insufficiency (Hurst, 1996).

Unique Identifier

Mother has implants in her breasts.

Ask yourself:
- Does the mother have nipple sensation? Did the surgery alter her sensation?
- Are the ducts patent?
- Are the nipple pores patent?
- Did the mother report any changes in breast size and/or appearance during pregnancy?

Watch out for:
- Engorgement and tight bras that can decrease milk supply.
- Insufficient milk.

What to do about it:
- Use tank tops with shelf bras for the first week or two to avoid pressure against the breast.
- Encourage the mother to report the surgery to the pediatric healthcare provider.

Expected resolution:
- Most women with breast implants have happy breastfeeding experiences.

What else to consider:
- Women sometimes need reassurance that breastfeeding will not harm their implants.
- Ask the mother about breast surgery when she is alone. Her partner and family members may not be aware of her surgery.
- Women may not think of this procedure as "surgery." We have come to ask women if they have had any "breast improvements."

In Our Opinion

It is important to have weekly (or more frequent) weight checks of the baby for the first months to ensure that there is adequate milk.

CONCERN: HISTORY OF BREAST SURGERY/INJURY

Descriptor: Breast Reduction

Women who have had breast reduction have a greater chance of lactation insufficiency and are more likely to stop full and overall breastfeeding sooner than women who have not (Souto, Giugliani, Giugliani, & Schneider, 2003).

Unique Identifier

Mother has had surgery to make her breasts smaller.

Ask yourself:
- Does the mother have sensation, especially down to her nipples? Did the surgery alter her sensation?
- Are the ducts patent?
- Are the nipple pores patent?
- Did the mother report any changes in breast size and/or appearance during pregnancy?

Watch out for:
- Adequacy of ongoing milk supply. Milk volume may increase around the third day; however, the nerves that convey sensation to the pituitary and signal adequate hormone release may have been severed or altered by surgery, and mature milk production may not be sustained at an adequate level.
- Insufficient milk-making tissue.
- Inability of milk to exit the breast because of severed ducts.
- Initial engorgement that does not resolve easily. This can be due to severed ducts, and may further reduce milk production.

What to do about it:
- Assessment and close follow-up with frequent weight checks in the first month and beyond.
- Ensure adequate nutrition for the baby.
- Consider at-breast supplementation if needed.
- Encourage the mother to report the surgery to the pediatric healthcare provider.

Expected resolution:
- There is no way to know ahead of time how much milk a mother will be able to make after breast reduction surgery. Frequent weight checks of the baby are mandatory throughout the first month and beyond.

What else to consider:
- Ask the mother about breast surgery when she is alone. Her partner and family members may not be aware of her surgery.
- Women may not think of this procedure as "surgery." We have come to ask women if they have had any "breast improvements."

In Our Opinion

It is important to have weekly (or more frequent) weight checks of the baby for the first month and beyond to ensure that there is adequate milk.

BREAST AND NIPPLE ISSUES

CONCERN: FLAT/INVERTED NIPPLE

Descriptor: Flat Nipple

Unique Identifier

Nipple appears level with surrounding tissue.

Ask yourself:

- Does the nipple evert (as in **Figure 6-1**)? (Using the asymmetric latch, the configuration of the nipple prior to latch is relatively unimportant. The concern is only if the nipple does not evert in the baby's mouth, because milk-making hormones may not be adequately released.)
- Is this a flat-appearing nipple (as in **Figure 6-2**) because it is stretched and occluded by engorgement?
  - Does the mother report that this is a new appearance for the nipple?
  - Is the area around the nipple engorged?
  - Is there pitting edema around the nipple?
- If the nipple was flat prior to the baby's birth, does the mother report that the nipple responds to cold or tactile stimulation by becoming more evert? If so, the nipple should respond easily when stimulated during breastfeeding.
- Is the baby able to compress the areola and breast tissue and draw the nipple area into the mouth to form the teat?

Watch out for:

- Mother's misunderstanding that the baby latches only to the nipple. Rather, baby forms a "teat" of nipple, areola, and some breast tissue.
- Thinking that a nipple has to look like a bottle nipple in order to work.
- Considering this to be a permanent situation.
- Flat nipple "epidemics" that are a result of poor maternity breastfeeding management practices (e.g., muscle relaxants used during labor, edema from excess fluids during labor).

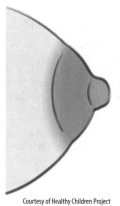

Courtesy of Healthy Children Project

Figure 6-1 The everted nipple protrudes out from the areola.

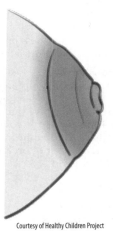

Courtesy of Healthy Children Project

Figure 6-2 The flat nipple everts when cold or manually stimulated.

BREAST AND NIPPLE ISSUES

- Confusing flat with inverted nipples (inverted nipples are drawn back into the breast).

What to do about it:
- If the mother reports that her nipple was flat before the baby was born, use the asymmetric latch technique described in Section 3. When the baby's bottom lip and jaw reach the breast first, the configuration of the flat nipple is unimportant.
- Document whether the nipple has everted during breastfeeding. We do this by standing behind the mother and observing the nipple at the moment of latch-off.
- If the nipple is flat because the nipple is engulfed within milk-filled tissue, hand expression or engorgement relief is needed so that the area is soft enough for the baby to draw into the mouth. Then use the asymmetric latch.

Expected resolution:
- Often, formerly flat nipples become everted over time with breastfeeding.
- Breastfeeding should not be a problem if flat nipples are managed appropriately.

What else to consider:
- Rarely, temporary use of a nipple shield may be appropriate for one or two feedings. (Long-term shield use may have negative ramifications on milk supply.) To use properly, follow the manufacturer's instructions for applying the shield so that an adequate amount of breast tissue is drawn into the tip of the shield.

In Our Opinion

Preventing engorgement and using the asymmetric latch are the keys to managing breastfeeding with flat nipples.

CONCERN: FLAT/INVERTED NIPPLE

Descriptor: Inverted Nipple

Unique Identifier

Nipple appears drawn into the surrounding tissue, as in **Figure 6-3**.

Ask yourself:

- Is this a nipple inverted by engorgement?
  - ○ Does the mother report that this is a new appearance for the nipple?
  - ○ Is the area around the nipple engorged?
  - ○ Is there pitting edema around the nipple?
- If the nipple was inverted prior to the baby's birth, does the mother report that the nipple responds to cold or tactile stimulation by becoming more erect?

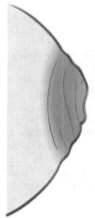

Courtesy of Healthy Children Project

Figure 6-3 The inverted nipple looks like a slit or a fold that should be graded by function, not appearance.

- Is the baby able to compress the areola and breast tissue and draw the nipple area into the mouth to form the teat?
- What grade is the inverted nipple? Remember that the grading system is about function not appearance (Han & Hong, 1999).
  - Grade 1 inverted nipples are easily pulled out by suckling or a breast pump.
  - Grade 2 inverted nipples are easily pulled out by suckling or a breast pump but don't maintain the projection once the baby's mouth leaves the nipple or the pump flange is removed.
  - Grade 3 inverted nipples are difficult or impossible to pull out. Some think that this is because there are internal breast anomalies, such as short ducts, associated with grade 3 nipples.

Watch out for:
- Prenatal nipple manipulations are not effective for inverted nipples and may cause mothers to give up breastfeeding sooner.
- Confusing flat with inverted nipples (inverted nipples are drawn back into the breast).
- Milk-supply problems. Women with inverted nipples have been shown to have less milk and lower prolactin levels in research studies (Aono, Shioku, Shoda, & Kurachi, 1977), and their babies have a higher risk of readmission for failure to thrive (Cooper, Atherton, Kahana, & Kotagal, 1995).
- Use the asymmetric latch technique described in Section 3. When the baby's bottom lip and jaw reach the breast first, the configuration of the nipple is less important.

What to do about it:
- Ask the mother if her nipple ever everts. If so, does she have a technique that will draw out the nipple? Can she do this prior to latching the baby to the breast?

- Document whether the nipple has everted during the breastfeeding. We do this by standing behind the mother and observing the nipple at the moment of latch-off.
- Ensure adequate nutrition for the baby. Some babies will suck happily even though the nipple is not drawn out. Remember, calorically deprived babies often act sleepy and satisfied.
- Encourage the mother to report this challenge to the pediatric healthcare provider to help assure close follow-up of baby's growth.

Expected resolution:
- Often, grade 1 and 2 nipples become everted over time with breastfeeding, hand expression, or pumping.
- In this situation, mothers will need to express milk as an adjunct to breastfeeding.
- With grade 3 nipples, there is a very high risk of milk insufficiency and failure to thrive. Frequent weight checks and diaper checks (Appendix I) and assessment of milk transfer (Appendix L) are necessary.
- Provide close ongoing pediatric follow-up to assess growth.

What else to consider:
- Some mothers find that using a hard plastic shell inside the bra in between feedings helps to dry and evert the nipple.
- Using a nipple shield with inverted nipples may further reduce the milk supply and put the baby at increased risk for failure to thrive. A milk expression plan is required to maintain milk supply if a shield is used.
- Calorically deprived babies act sleepy. The baby sleeping more and acting content is an ominous sign. Frequent weight checks are the only way to know how the baby is doing with breastfeeding if there is an inverted nipple.

In Our Opinion

Inverted nipples are related to failure to thrive and readmission for hypernatremic dehydration and malnutrition in the baby. Assessment of the breastfeeding (Appendix B), assessment of milk transfer (Appendix L), and frequent weight checks are necessary with inverted nipples, but are especially important with grade 3 inverted nipples.

CONCERN: NIPPLE PAIN WHILE BREASTFEEDING (FIGURE 6-4)

Descriptor: Nipple Pain While the Baby Is Latched On and Actively Nursing

Nipple pain may be common, but it is not normal. Any pain that a mother experiences should be thoroughly investigated. Nipple pain while the baby is actively feeding may be:

- Worse at the beginning of the nursing.
- Continuous throughout the nursing.
  - Beginning in the first few days.
  - Beginning after there is an abundant amount of milk (day 3 or 4 onward).

Unique Identifier

Intense nipple pain that is worse at the beginning, for the first minute or two, and then subsides or continues at a lower level.

Ask yourself:
- Is the baby latching on suboptimally and then correcting his or her head or body position to accommodate a better flow of milk?
- Does a change in position or body motion coincide with the change in pain level?

Watch out for:
- Baby head change, body movement, or other changes as the pain level decreases.

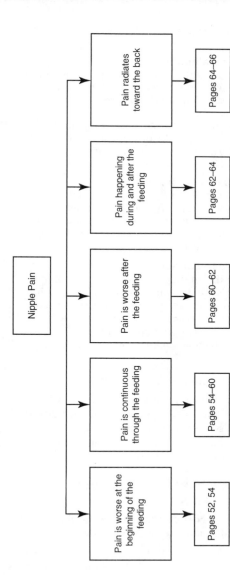

Figure 6-4 Nipple pain.

53

What to do about it:
- Watch the baby nursing, paying close attention to the change in the baby's sucking, head position, and mother's posture the instant the pain level changes.
- Position the baby in the new (less painful) position to begin the next feeding. The mother should become attentive to positioning the baby in the pain-free position.

Expected resolution:
- Although there may be some residual pain for a day or so if the nipple has been damaged, the mother's pain level should markedly decrease with more optimal positioning from the beginning of the feeding.

What else to consider:
- During the feeding, carefully examine the mother's fingers, hand, or arm. Is she putting pressure against the back of the baby's head? If so, this may cause the baby to pull back, stretching the nipple uncomfortably.
- Could it be that a pillow is changing the angle of the baby's head?

In Our Opinion

Nipple creams and other treatments will not fix this problem. In fact, the use of these commonly used preparations may discourage the mother from seeking help and working on corrective positioning interventions.

CONCERN: NIPPLE PAIN WHILE BREASTFEEDING

Descriptor: Nipple Pain While the Baby Is Latched On and Actively Nursing

Nipple pain is common, but it is not normal. Any pain experienced by the mother should be thoroughly investigated. Nipple pain while the baby is actively feeding may be:

- Worse at the beginning of the nursing.
- Continuous throughout the nursing:
  - Beginning in the first few days.
  - Beginning after there is an abundant amount of milk (day 3 or 4 onward).

Unique Identifier

Nipple pain that begins in the first few days and continues throughout the nursing. Nipple that is misshapen when the baby latches off. A compression line may be visible, as in **Figure 6-5**. The baby may spit up blood-tinged milk, or the mother may express milk colored by small drops of blood.

Ask yourself:

- Did the soreness start before there was an abundant supply of milk?
- Is the nipple misshapen after the baby comes off of the breast?

If yes, consider:

- Suboptimal position of the baby at the breast.

What to do about it:

- Assess the next breastfeed, including the prefeeding behaviors using the breastfeeding assessment criteria in Appendix B.
- Use corrective interventions to optimize the latching process and positioning for the feeding.
- If blood is seen, reassure the mother that her blood will not harm the baby.

Expected resolution:

- Although there may be some residual pain for a day or so if the nipple has been damaged, the mother's pain level should improve dramatically with more optimal positioning

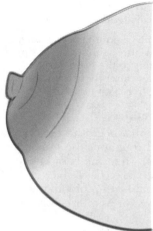

Courtesy of Healthy Children Project

Figure 6-5 Suboptimal latch may cause nipple compression.

(Cadwell, Turner-Maffei, Blair, Brimdyr, & McInerney, 2004).
- If the baby has been positioned optimally, the nipple will not be misshapen after the baby latches off the breast.

What else to consider:
- Correcting the position will markedly decrease the pain for more than 95 percent of dyads.
- A few babies exert higher than average amounts of pressure at the breast; others may have palate shapes that require persistent corrective measures. The arrival of abundant milk flow may encourage some babies to decrease pressure. The mother may use "breast compression" or "alternate massage" to increase milk flow and to diminish pressure (Appendix D).

- "Tongue tie" may be associated with continuous sore nipples. Many mothers have reported relief after the frenulum stretches or has been divided by a qualified healthcare provider.
  ○ Palate configurations that are a result of "molding" or "caput" of the infant's skull usually resolve over time. If close follow-up of mother and baby is possible, consider temporary use of a nipple shield, while protecting milk supply, if the baby has a high palate.

Research confirms that:
- Positioning the baby correctly is effective in diminishing pain for almost every mother (Cadwell et al., 2004).

CONCERN: NIPPLE PAIN WHILE BREASTFEEDING

Descriptor: Oversupply

Nipple pain is common, but it is not normal. Nipple pain while the baby is actively feeding may be:

- Worse at the beginning.
- Continuous:
  ○ Beginning during the first few days.
  ○ Beginning after there is an abundant amount of milk (day 3 or 4 onward).

Unique Identifier

Nipple pain that begins after there is an abundant supply of milk and continues throughout each nursing. Nipple is misshapen when the baby latches off. This may be the constellation of factors called "oversupply."

Ask yourself:
- Is the pain worse after the first few days?
- Does the mother have an abundant supply of milk?

BREAST AND NIPPLE ISSUES

- Do the mother and baby have any other signs of "oversupply"?

Consider:
- Sometimes a baby can manage the slower flow of colostrum but has trouble managing the abundant and rapid flow of milk after day 3 or 4.
- The pain may be related to the baby clamping down on the nipple because the flow of milk is too abundant or too rapid for the baby to handle.
- The problem of oversupply often has a constellation of findings, including rapid weight gain of the baby and many large explosive bowel movements (comes out of diaper), along with the pain during feedings that usually causes the mother to ask for help. The baby is often unsettled after feeding and may spit up or vomit a quantity of milk.
- Considering that the baby is gaining well, the baby may still not act contented between feedings, giving the mother the mistaken idea that she does not have enough milk or that there is "something wrong" with her milk.
- Weights taken before and after nursing with a digital scale accurate to 2 grams show rapid transfer of more than expected amounts of milk at the breast in a shorter than expected amount of time (for example, 3 ounces in 5 minutes in a baby under 1 month of age). (See Appendix E for the before and after weight protocol.)

What to do about it:
- Help the mother achieve a posture in which the baby is able to move his or her head freely when the flow of milk is too great or too fast to handle (Appendix K).
- One position that works well is where the mother is reclining or semireclining (see Figure C-4 in Appendix C) and the baby's body is supported on the mother's. The mother is "down under" the

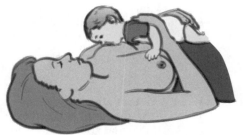

Courtesy of Healthy Children Project

Figure 6-6 When using the Australian posture, the mother is "down under."

baby (as in **Figure 6-6**), which is why this is called the Australian posture, and the baby no longer has to work against the milk flow.
- More aggressive treatment may include nursing on only one breast at each feeding to allow a small amount of breast compression to tamp back the supply. A firm, but not overly tight, bra may also help. The mother must be careful not to allow too much pressure because that could foster mastitis.
- Massive oversupply may respond to nursing on the same breast for two or more feedings in a row. Again, watch for plugged ducts and mastitis.
- Instead of decreasing the milk supply using compression, some mothers prefer to collect the extra milk and donate to a mothers' milk bank. See Appendix Y for donation information.

Expected resolution:
- Although there may be some residual pain for a day or so if the nipple has been damaged, the mother's pain level should disappear with the baby in control of the flow rather than overwhelmed by it.
- The nipple should not be distorted after nursing.

What else to consider:

- Excessive hand expression or pumping to get rid of the "extra" milk may compound the problem by relieving the compression on the cells. As a result, the milk supply continues to increase.

In Our Opinion

For many years, poor breastfeeding management practices highlighted the issue of "not enough breastmilk." We think that the constellation of oversupply of breastmilk is increasingly common as more and more mothers choose to breastfeed, and breastfeed exclusively and for longer durations. It seems to be more likely to happen with second or subsequent breastfed babies.

CONCERN: NIPPLE AND BREAST PAIN AFTER BREASTFEEDING

Descriptor: Raynaud's Phenomenon (Vasospasm) of the Nipple

Nipple pain is common, but it is not normal. Any nipple pain should be investigated thoroughly.

Unique Identifier

Excruciating nipple and breast pain after nursing and at other times when the nipple is cold or wet; always accompanied by nipple color change (waxy white, quickly transient to cyanotic blue, and then to raspberry pink, or white to pink). Often the areola changes shape at the same time.

- Pain is worse after the nursing/pumping/hand expression.
- Although the mother may describe the greatest amount of pain near the nipple, pain may radiate throughout the breast.

- The mother also may experience pain if the nipples are cold and/or wet, when getting out of the shower, for example.
- The pain is excruciating (mother may describe the pain as burning or stabbing).
- Consider a diagnosis of nipple vasospasm, or Raynaud's phenomenon of the nipple.

Ask yourself:
- Does the nipple look white and waxy seconds to minutes after the baby comes off the breast? After pumping? After showering? When cold/wet?
- Is the pain related to the nipple changing from being warm to being cold?
- Does drying/warming the nipple and breast decrease the pain?

Watch out for:
- Confusing this with "yeast" (*Candida albicans*) problems. Nipples do not turn white if the problem is yeast (although white patches may be seen in the baby's mouth). Also, if the problem is yeast, the mother usually describes the pain as burning, during and after the feeding. The nipple and areolar skin is usually shiny with flaking if the problem is yeast (Francis-Morrill, Heinig, Pappagianis, & Dewey, 2004).

What to do about it:
- Ensure optimal positioning.
- Eliminate any other causes of painful nipples that can contribute to nipple pain. Sometimes mothers keep warmed cloths nearby to warm their nipple after feeding so that the nipple cools more slowly.
- Nifedipine has been prescribed for nursing mothers with Raynaud's symptoms of the nipples with good results (Anderson, Held, & Wright, 2004).

BREAST AND NIPPLE ISSUES

Expected resolution:
- Some mothers report a marked reduction in pain once the cause of nipple vasospasm has been corrected, but nifedipine may also be considered. In our experience with mothers taking nifedipine, it may take several days of treatment for the pain to resolve completely.

What else to consider:
- Raynaud's can happen simultaneously with suboptimal positioning, high mouth pressure during suck, nipple infection, eczema, and other breast and nipple conditions. Each possibility should be considered.

In Our Experience

We have seen mothers who had Raynaud's symptoms of their nipples from their early teens. Often, there is a family history of Raynaud's. One mother told us that she was surprised that anyone liked to swim because she assumed that everybody had painful nipples after swimming. We have also seen mothers who developed Raynaud's after a long course of painful and infected nipples.

CONCERN: NIPPLE/BREAST PAIN WHILE BREASTFEEDING AND CONTINUING AFTER AND BETWEEN FEEDINGS

Descriptor: *Candida Albicans,* Yeast or Thrush

Unique Identifier

Burning pain during and after breastfeeding. Shiny, flaky skin is visible on the nipple and areola in more than 90 percent of cases (Francis-Morrill et al., 2004). In addition, white patches are usually seen in the baby's mouth inside the cheeks and on the tongue. The baby's diaper area may also have a yeast rash.

Ask yourself:
- Has the mother had antibiotic treatment that would predispose her to *C. albicans* overgrowth?
- Are the positioning and latch optimal? (Appendix B)

Watch out for:
- Overdiagnosis of yeast as the cause of sore nipples without consideration of other possibilities.
- Confusing this stabbing pain with yeast inside the breast. Hale, Bateman, Finkelman, and Berens (2009) found no *C. albicans in* the milk of women with deep breast pain, and suggest that it does not migrate into the breast. Research indicates that this condition is most likely to be associated with bacterial infection (Thomassen, Johansson, Wassberg, & Petrini, 1998).

What to do about it:
- Mother, baby, and any vectors must be treated. Vectors can include breast pump parts, pacifiers, bottle nipples, and any other object that can harbor *C. albicans*. In some cases, another family member may harbor *C. albicans*. Treatment is only effective when the vector has also been eliminated.
- A variety of treatments are available to be prescribed for both mother and baby. For example, the oral suspension nystatin may be carefully applied inside the baby's mouth, being sure to coat all surfaces. Nystatin may also be applied to the mother's nipple, her areola, and the baby's mouth. Fluconazole, an oral medication used to treat *C. albicans,* may be prescribed for both mother and baby.
- In addition, breast pump parts, washable breast pads, bras, and other possible vectors should be carefully cleaned. The usual recommendation is to boil any components that touch the skin or the milk for 20 minutes.
- Pacifiers are best discarded.

Expected resolution:
- If the treatment is effective and vectors are effectively cleaned, the mother should begin to feel relief in 1 or 2 days. It may take 5 to 14 days to finish prescriptions. The mother should report progress in pain reduction.

What else to consider:
- Deep, radiating breast pain is more likely to be related to a bacterial rather than to *C. albicans* (Thomassen et al., 1998).
- There is a concern about yeast in stored/frozen milk. Freezing does not kill yeast. This is less of a concern for older, healthy babies than it is for premies or for fragile or ill babies.

In Our Opinion

We have seen many cases of mothers who have come to the Center for Breastfeeding with "persistent" cases of breast and nipple "yeast" without symptoms in the baby. The problem for virtually every one of these mothers was actually suboptimal latch and positioning. Yeast treatments had been instituted without a careful evaluation of latch and positioning. The yeast treatments were thought to be ineffective because the soreness did not lessen. Always assess latch-on and positioning, even in cases where visible yeast is present.

CONCERN: NIPPLE PAIN THAT RADIATES THROUGH THE BREAST AND EVEN TO THE BACK

Descriptor: Bleb (Sometimes Called a Milk Blister)

Unique Identifier

A firm, small, white spot ("bleb," or duct blocked near the nipple pore opening) of accumulated milk solids visible on the nipple face.

Sometimes the nipple itself may be distended, especially if there are multiple blocked nipple pores. Occasionally, nipple skin "grows over" the bleb and prevents the bleb's removal without lancing.

The mother experiences nipple pain while the baby is latched on and actively nursing as well as between feedings. Pain usually also increases when anything (such as clothing) touches the breast and radiates from the nipple tip toward the mother's back.

Ask yourself:
- Can the baby extract the retained milk with more effective feeding?

Watch out for:
- Reoccurrence if the underlying problem is not addressed.
- The development of systemic symptoms (fever, malaise) that may indicate onset of mastitis.

What to do about it:
- Work with the mother to achieve a more effective position.
- Will soaking the breast in warm water prior to nursing or hand expression help to "loosen" the bleb?
- Will gentle hand expression and finger manipulation expel the bleb?
- Has skin (or a clear layer of tissue) accumulated over the bleb? Is that the reason the bleb is not moving out of the nipple? In some cases, lancing followed by expression of the retained milk is the only way to solve the problem. The milk behind the bleb is usually thick (the consistency of softened cream cheese). A few drops of blood are not unusual after lancing.
- Why did the bleb form? Is part of the breast draining poorly? Tight bra? Underwire? Other

constriction on milk flow? Bruise? Was there a plugged duct further up in the breast prior to the bleb forming?

Expected resolution:
- Once the bleb and the milk behind it are removed, the pain should decrease markedly.

What else to consider:
- Plugged ducts.
- Mastitis (will have systemic symptoms).

In Our Opinion

No one really understands why some women get blebs. There are reports of women with repetitive cases of plugged ducts or blebs who increase the amount of lecithin in their diets and have some success in reducing their incidence. We have known mothers for whom this has worked.

CONCERN: SWOLLEN, PAINFUL BREASTS

Descriptor: Engorgement

Unique Identifier

Painfully swollen breasts, as in **Figure 6-7**, often between days 2 and 4 after birth, or later if the baby was born via cesarean section. This can also happen any time in the early weeks if the baby is not feeding often or effectively enough.

Ask yourself:
- Is the baby feeding frequently and efficiently enough? (Appendices B and E)
- Is the baby positioned well at the breast? (Appendix B)
- Is there a mild fever without an area of redness on the breast?

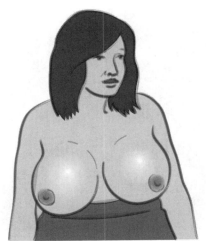

Courtesy of Healthy Children Project

Figure 6-7 When the breasts are engorged they are hard and hot. The skin may be so stretched that it is shiny.

Watch out for:
- Redness, malaise, flu-like symptoms—signs of mastitis.

What to do about it:
- Increase frequency and efficiency of breastfeedings.
- Relieve pressure and pain by allowing excess milk to flow out of the breast. Water is a wonderful aid: Either the shower or bath, or breast water baths (as in **Figure 6-8**), may help the milk flow and relieve compression.
- The mother should allow the baby to nurse until he or she comes off spontaneously. If the baby is not interested in taking the second breast at that feeding, offer that breast first the next time cues are seen (often within a half hour in the first days).

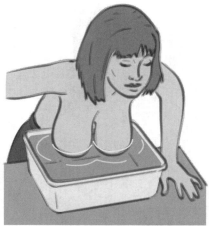

Courtesy of Healthy Children Project

Figure 6-8 Lukewarm water (in this case in a dishpan) helps to relieve engorgement by encouraging milk to flow.

- Gentle expression may also relieve pressure.
- Consider mild analgesics, especially if they are also nonsteroidal anti-inflammatory (NSAID) medications.

Expected resolution:
- Improving frequency and efficiency of feedings, along with relief of some pressure, should decrease the pain and discomfort within hours. It may take a few days for the engorgement to completely resolve.

What else to consider:
- The natural swelling in the breast beginning on days 2 through 4 is not only because of accumulated milk. There is an increased amount of blood and lymph that will resolve as the days pass.

- Suboptimal breastfeeding increases the amount of milk, leading to engorgement. Almost all mothers experience "normal fullness" without high levels of pain and discomfort.

Evidence-based review of the literature:
- Does not support either warm or cold applications as the superior choice in the relief of engorgement. Mothers may feel comforted by either, and each mother should choose comfort measures based on cultural belief (exposure to cold during the postpartum period is not considered healthful in many cultures).
- Does not support the use of cabbage leaves or cabbage salves over cool gel packs or other comfort measures for reducing pain and engorgement (Mangesi & Dowswell, 2010). The best possible method to reduce engorgement is to keep the milk flowing and the baby nursing effectively.

In Our Experience

We have seen rare cases where the engorgement resolves in only one breast; the other continues to be swollen with pitting edema. This does not seem to be an issue with milk, but rather with lymph drainage. Techniques to promote lymph drainage (e.g., exercise, massage) have been helpful in the successful resolution of this residual swelling.

CONCERN: BREAST LUMPS

Descriptor: Plugged Duct; Also Called Clogged Duct or Caked Breast

Unique Identifier

Hard, (often) painful area of the breast, swollen (plugged or clogged) with milk because of temporarily poor milk drainage but with no systemic symptoms.

Ask yourself:
- How can positioning and milk transfer be improved?

Watch out for:
- Are there any systemic symptoms (e.g., fever, malaise)? If any are present, consider that this could be mastitis.
- Is the skin over the hard, painful area reddened? Again, consider that this could be mastitis.

What to do about it:
- Have the mother give an accurate description of the plug's location. For example, "right breast, 11 o'clock, four finger widths from the base of the nipple." That way, it can be documented how the lump has moved.
- Consider encouraging the mother to start on the side with the plug to maximize flow when the baby's suckling is the most efficient.
- Change posture (and the baby's body position). Changing position at the breast may allow the plug to exit the breast. Many mothers find that changing position so that the baby's chin points in another direction at the breast is helpful.
- Gentle massage during breastfeeding on the affected side may move the plug toward the nipple.

Expected resolution:
- The plug should move toward the nipple with each feeding and disappear within 24 to 48 hours.
- Tenderness in the area of the lump may be reported for several days after the lump has moved.
- The lump may come out as stringy milk or a hardened blob of milk. This is not harmful for the baby to consume. Occasionally, dried milk solids lodge in the nipple as blebs.

What else to consider:
- Lumps in the breast can have many other causes; if the plugs do not move out in 24 to 48 hours, a physical exam by a qualified healthcare provider is required.

In Our Opinion

Blocked ducts tend to happen when the breast is not draining as well as it should. Careful assessment of a feeding, and examination of possible clothing compression on the breast can help determine the underlying reason for the development of the plug, and correction may serve to prevent or minimize future plugs.

CONCERN: REDDENED AREA OF BREAST WITH SYSTEMIC SYMPTOMS

Descriptor: Mastitis

Unique Identifier

The mother suddenly feels ill with flu-like symptoms and has a painful, hard, reddened area on one breast. Mastitis always indicates inflammation in the breast and may be either infective or noninfective.

Ask yourself:
- Could the mother be ill with something besides mastitis? Other causes for the symptoms should be considered.

Watch out for:
- Are both breasts reddened with fever and flu-like symptoms? If so, this is a potential medical emergency (e.g., strep infection) for which the mother should seek care urgently.
- Mastitis that is not treated promptly and effectively may result in abscess.

What to do about it:
- Mastitis may be infective or noninfective, but it always indicates an inflammatory process. Consider nonsteroidal anti-inflammatory (NSAID) medications.
- If improved breastfeeding practices and NSAID medications do not resolve the symptoms, or if the symptoms become worse in a few hours, consider a course of antibiotics if infection is suspected (for example, if there are nipple fissures or signs of nipple damage). *Staphylococcus aureus* is the most likely organism cultured in cases of infective mastitis, although a variety of other organisms have been implicated.
- Think about the cause of mastitis and how to decrease the chance of mastitis recurring. According to Fetherston (1998) and Amir, Forster, Lumley, and McLachlan (2007), predictive factors for mastitis include:
  ○ Ineffective, hurried feedings.
  ○ Plugged ducts.
  ○ Suboptimal feedings.
  ○ Tight bra, underwire bra, or pressure on the breast.
  ○ Nipple damage.
  ○ Anemic mothers (especially if mastitis is recurrent).
  ○ Use of breast shell inside the bra between feedings, or nipple shield during feedings.
  ○ Short lingual frenulum or "tongue-tied" baby.
- Help the mother think about taking care of herself (bed rest, fever reduction, and NSAID) and improving breastfeeding practices. Breastfeed frequently. Mastitis, even infective mastitis, does not require breastfeeding suspension or cessation.

Expected resolution:
- Symptoms should resolve in 5 days, usually before the prescribed antibiotic is finished. Encourage the mother to continue taking the

antibiotic (if prescribed) even after the symptoms resolve.

What else to consider:
- Anemia in the case of recurrent mastitis.
- Inflammatory breast cancer.

In Our Experience

Mothers feel as though they have been "run over by a truck," when mastitis hits. Prompt medical attention, rest, and appropriate changes to breastfeeding practices result in speedy recovery for most mothers. There is no need to interrupt breastfeeding.

Breast cancer diagnosis, especially diagnosis of inflammatory breast cancer, may be delayed in breastfeeding mothers because of the mistaken diagnosis of recurrent mastitis. Breast cancer, including inflammatory breast cancer and Paget's disease of the breast, have been diagnosed in the population of currently breastfeeding mothers.

CONCERN: BREAST LUMP WITH FLU-LIKE SYMPTOMS

Descriptor: Abscess

Unique Identifier

Pus-filled lump in the breast that does not move. Abscess is often associated with continuation of mastitis symptoms after 5 days of appropriate antibiotic treatment, but may occur without a history of mastitis. The affected area of the breast is usually tender.

Ask yourself:
- Is the tender lump milk or pus? Needle aspiration is needed to confirm the diagnosis.

Watch out for:
- The worst solution is to stop breastfeeding/ milk expression altogether or even stopping only on the affected side. Suddenly stopping breastfeeding will make the problem worse; engorgement will become part of the problem.
- If the choice is made to "dry up" on the affected breast, it should be done slowly.
- Pus may drain out through the nipple; this will relieve some of the pressure but does not preclude medical treatment. Do not put pressure on a draining abscess.
- The possibility of methycillin-resistant *Staphylococcus aureus* (MRSA) infection in the abscess. This appears to be on the rise (Branch-Elliman et al., 2012; Montalto & Lui, 2009; Stafford et al., 2008).

What to do about it:
- Refer the mother to her obstetric care provider, who can assess the need for:
  - Evaluation for abscess. Usually diagnosis is confirmed by needle aspiration of pus. (Ultrasound may indicate fluid but may not sufficiently differentiate between abscess and galactocele.)
  - Drainage or surgical removal of the abscess. Repeated needle aspiration is sometimes successful. The newer technique is to insert a drain (or drains) using ultrasound to guide the placement (Christensen et al., 2005). Often, surgery is performed in an outpatient setting with local anesthesia. The incision should be made as far away from the nipple and areola as possible. Every attempt should be made to avoid cutting across ducts.
  - Antibiotic therapy and nonsteroidal anti-inflammatory, fever-reducing medications.
- After diagnosis and treatment:
  - Recommend bed rest and continued breast-feeding on the unaffected side.

○ Encourage continued breastfeeding on the affected side if possible. If putting the baby to breast is not possible, hand expression or gentle pumping should be recommended to remove milk.

○ Assess breastfeeding and ensure that any pressure on the breast that might hinder milk flow is removed.

Expected resolution:
- The abscess will be removed and the area healed.
- Breastfeeding can definitely continue on the unaffected breast, and, at a minimum, milk supply should be maintained until the baby can return to the breast that had the abscess.

What else to consider:
- Galactocele.
- Breast cancer.

In Our Opinion

Abscesses happen rarely, but they are usually the result of untreated or inadequately treated plugged ducts or mastitis.

SECTION 7

Breastfeeding Management Issues

WHEN TO BREASTFEED:
FEEDING FREQUENCY

It's hard to predict how many times a day a breastfed baby will be fed, when fed "on demand." Some mothers wish they could know how long their baby can go between nursings. There are several factors that come into play when determining a range in feeding frequency for a breastfed infant.

- Mothers have different amounts of "storage capacity" in their breasts. This is the amount of milk that can accumulate before giving the mammary cells the message to make less milk. One mother may have a storage capacity that allows the breasts to go longer or shorter between feedings compared with another mother.
- Babies have a range of skill in latching and transferring milk. The more opportunities the baby has to practice breastfeeding, the more skill he or she will develop.
- Calorically deprived babies are sleepy and apathetic feeders. Sometimes, mothers and caregivers can mistake a sleepy, poorly nourished, calorically deprived baby for a contented baby.
- Breastmilk is perfect for the human baby; it is very easy to digest. That means that breastmilk needs to be fed more frequently than nonhuman foods, such as formula.
- Crying babies may shut down at the breast and look as if they are asleep when they have actually given up.

- Newborn breastfed babies need to nurse 10 to 12 times a day.
- Many people have come to think of the baby crying as the signal to begin a breastfeeding. Crying is actually a very late feeding signal. By the time babies cry, they have often become disorganized and do not feed as well.

Feeding Cues

Feeding cues are signs that the baby is in a state that is favorable to feeding. These signs begin during periods of active sleep (identified by the presence of rapid eye movement [REM] in the baby). As the baby becomes hungrier and more awake, feeding cues become more obvious. The baby begins to bring his or her fist to the mouth; to seek food with the lips, tongue, and head; to smack the lips or extend the tongue; and so on. Feeding cues include:

- Rooting—turning the head, especially with searching movements of the mouth, as in **Figure 7-1**.

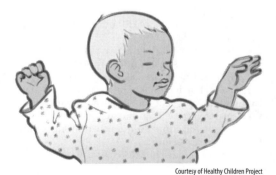

Courtesy of Healthy Children Project

Figure 7-1 Subtle body motions are a feeding cue.

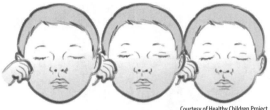

Courtesy of Healthy Children Project

Figure 7-2 Rapid eye movement (REM) is a feeding cue.

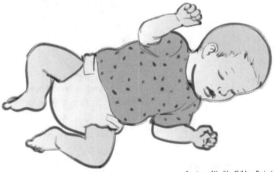

Courtesy of Healthy Children Project

Figure 7-3 Body motions, including flexing of the arms and legs, are feeding cues.

- Increasing alertness, especially REM under closed eyelids, as in **Figure 7-2**.
- Flexing of the legs and arms, as in **Figure 7-3**.
- Attempting to bring a hand to the mouth, as in **Figure 7-4**.
- Sucking on a fist or finger.
- Mouthing motions of the lips and tongue, as in Figure 7-4.
- Crying is considered a late feeding cue because it does not usually begin in intact, full-term infants until more subtle cues have failed to elicit the mother's attention.

MANAGEMENT ISSUES

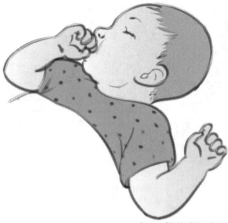

Courtesy of Healthy Children Project

Figure 7-4 Putting the hand near or in the mouth is a feeding cue.

Less mature and more disorganized infants may pass quickly from the state of deep sleep (characterized by no REM) to crying. Skin-to-skin holding can help infants with motor-state maturation. An infant who is showing subtle feeding cues should be held skin to skin between feedings.

EXPECTED WEIGHT GAIN IN THE BREASTFED BABY

- After an initial weight loss of 7 percent or less, adequately nourished breastfed infants should have no further body weight loss by day 5 (AAP, 2012).
- After that, exclusively breastfed infants should gain 1 ounce or more a day, a more rapid gain

in the early months than is shown by the average baby on standardized growth charts. That's because the standard National Center for Health Statistics (NCHS) charts were developed using the combined growth averages of formula-fed, mixed-fed, and breastfed infants (Turner-Maffei & Cadwell, 2015). We now know that when only breastfed infants' weights are considered, they gain in a different pattern, growing more rapidly in the early months.

- At about 6 months, breastfed babies should begin eating solid foods.
- During the second half of the first year, breastfed babies, even if well fed, gain more slowly than formula-fed infants.
- The WHO growth curves should be used to monitor the growth of all children younger than 24 months, regardless of feeding method (AAP, 2012; Centers for Disease Control and Prevention [CDC], 2010).

WEIGHT LOSS IN THE NEWBORN

According to the American Academy of Pediatrics (AAP), weight loss in the newborn should be no more than 7 percent from birth weight.

- If a breastfeeding newborn has lost more than 7 percent of his or her birth weight (Appendix H), there should be prompt and intensive evaluation of breastfeeding.
- Interventions to correct problems and improve milk production and transfer should be initiated with careful follow-up.
- If breastfeeding problems cannot be identified and promptly corrected, ensure adequate nutrition for the infant with the mother's expressed milk, donor milk from an HMBANA (Appendix Y) or appropriately licensed milk bank, or appropriate breastmilk substitute.

MANAGEMENT ISSUES

INSUFFICIENT MILK

One of the critical issues surrounding the insufficient milk syndrome for clinicians is whether it is an actual problem of not enough milk or a *perceived* problem of not enough milk.

- Some mothers believe that colostrum is low in quantity and not sufficient for the baby. They may even want to start formula right away, even though they have plans to breastfeed later when there is a more abundant supply.
  - Colostrum is the ideal milk for newborn babies; it is rightly called "newborn milk."[1] Colostrum is high in antibodies and other components that begin to protect the baby from pathogens.
  - It is best if the baby has many opportunities to learn to breastfeed before the time of abundant milk.
- One might naïvely think that a fussy baby is a hungry baby and that a quiet baby is a full and content baby. Within the range of "normal," this may hold true, but underfed, calorically deprived babies begin to conserve energy, cry less, and sleep more. Unfortunately, this behavior may serve to reinforce the mother's behavior of restricting feeds.
- As the baby continues to be calorically deprived, the suck may weaken, further diminishing the stimulus required by the mother's breasts to continue producing an adequate supply of milk. This example demonstrates how a mother with an adequate milk supply may diminish her quantity of milk by unfortunate behavior she mistakenly believes will increase her milk supply.

---

[1]Thanks to our colleague, Nikki Lee, for this excellent description.

- There are two forms of milk insufficiency: *actual* and *perceived*. In the case of actual milk insufficiency, some mothers may be aware of the situation and perceive that there is inadequate milk. Other mothers may see their baby as more content, as the baby becomes more and more calorically deprived.
- Mothers may notice that they have insufficient milk when pumping. In this case, some ideas to consider include:
  - Starting with hand expression. Studies show that combining hand expression and pumping increases milk yield when compared with pumping alone (Flaherman et al., 2012; Morton et al., 2009) and may also increase caloric content of the milk collected (Morton et al., 2012).
  - Assessing the pumping:
    - Pump both sides at once.
    - Determine whether the pump is missing parts or not working properly.
    - Determine whether the flange is too tight. Many mothers need a larger flange (see Appendix Y for sources of larger sizes). If the nipple does not move freely inside the flange, the flange is probably too small. (Note: Sometimes it is obvious that a mother's nipple is too large for the flange. Other times, the smallish nipple swells during the pumping session. Watch her pumping to see if there is room for the nipple to be stretched inside the tunnel of the pump flange. If the tunnel is full of nipple and breast tissues, try a larger diameter flange.)
  - Trying guided imagery while expressing milk. The mother listens to an audio recording of a progressive relaxation, while imagining the ocean or a waterfall of milk (Feher, Berger, Johnson, & Wilde, 1989).

MANAGEMENT ISSUES

- ○ Trying power pumping. Instead of pumping for 15 minutes straight, for example, she might try pumping for a few minutes, stopping for a few minutes, then repeating. This may take longer than 15 minutes.
- ○ Trying a pump flange with a different shape. The ducts are right behind the nipple, so some flanges decrease the milk flow for some mothers the same way a baby with a clenched mouth can.
- ○ Trying a different style of pump. Some pumps use more compression and less vacuum.
- Many mothers who perceive they do not have enough milk actually have an adequate milk supply. Assessing the baby's growth using an appropriate growth chart or, if appropriate, calculating test weights (Appendix E) may be helpful in pointing out the baby's adequate growth to the parents.

MATERNAL REASONS FOR INADEQUATE MILK SUPPLY

Many reasons have been reported for mothers having an inadequate milk supply for their baby, as demonstrated by poor weight gain in the infant. (If the problem is inadequate pumped or expressed milk, please see the section on milk collection and storage.)

Consider:
- Inadequate breast stimulation (possible causes: inverted nipples that do not evert when stimulated, use of nipple shield without additional milk expression, etc.).
- Infrequent breastfeeding (scheduled feedings, use of formula or pacifiers to increase the time between feedings, etc.).
- Inadequate milk removal resulting in engorgement.

- Suboptimal hormone balance:
  - Retained placental fragments.
  - Hypothyroidism.
  - Hyperthyroidism.
  - Sheehan's syndrome (pituitary infarct).
  - Insulin (mothers with insulin-dependent diabetes mellitus [IDDM] may bring in an abundant milk supply later than mothers without diabetes).
  - Theca lutein cyst or polycystic ovarian syndrome (PCOS).
- Smoking (however, mothers who smoke should be encouraged to breastfeed).
- Breast injury.
- Congenital breast anomalies.
- Discrepancy in the size between a mother's breasts, which may be congenital or caused by injury or surgery (also known as "asymmetric breasts").
- Breast surgery.
- Certain drugs (e.g., pseudoephedrine [Hale, 2014], corticosteroids [Henderson, Hartmann, Newnham, & Simmer, 2008], early administration of birth control drugs) and high doses of vitamin B_6, which may delay lactogenesis.
- New pregnancy.
- Maternal depression (see tool for identifying women at risk for mood disorders in Appendix S).

Not related to decreased milk production:
- Maternal fluid intake (mothers should drink to avoid thirst, but drinking more fluid will not make more milk).
- Physical labor.
- Maternal stress (breastfeeding women are likely to experience less stress than those who are formula feeding [Groër, 2005]).
- Maternal "fatigue" without an underlying physical cause such as those listed.
- Maternal diet (malnourished women produce adequate milk).

MOTHER'S DIET

The breastmilk of mothers around the world, who eat very different diets from each other, is remarkably similar. Mothers do not need a balanced diet every day to make good milk. In fact, women who are starving and in famine have milk virtually identical to women who are well nourished and have been well nourished for their whole lives. However:

- Mothers who are well nourished have been found to play with their babies more than mothers who are not well nourished.
- Mothers who are well nourished are more likely to exclusively breastfeed longer than mothers who are not well nourished.
- Because of maternal physiologic changes and the use of maternal fat stores, mothers may require fewer than 500 additional calories a day while they are breastfeeding.

Thus, mothers who are breastfeeding should be encouraged to eat well for their own well-being, not with the idea that dietary choices will affect their breastmilk on a day-to-day basis.

Mothers' dietary choices:

- Convey the flavors of the culture to the baby by flavoring mothers' milk. Spicy and gassy foods should only be excluded on a case-by-case basis, not as a general rule.
- Babies seem to prefer flavored milk. In a research study, they nursed almost twice as long when the mother had eaten garlic (Beauchamp & Mennella, 2011).
- Babies seem to get used to the flavors in the mother's diet by swallowing amniotic fluid, which, like breastmilk, takes on the flavors of the mother's food (Mennella, Jagnow, & Beauchamp, 2001).

- Chocolate, coffee, tea, and diet sodas with caffeine can be enjoyed by nursing mothers in moderation.
- According to the Institute of Medicine, alcohol may be consumed in moderation by nursing mothers. If alcohol is used, advise the lactating woman to limit her intake to no more than 0.5 g of alcohol per kg of maternal body weight per day. For a 60-kg (132-pound) woman, 0.5 g of alcohol per kg of body weight corresponds to approximately 2 to 2.5 oz of liquor, 8 oz of table wine, or 2 cans of beer (Institute of Medicine, 1991).
- Colicky breastfed babies may be reacting to cow's milk whey in their mother's diet. It may take 10 days to 2 weeks of eliminating liquid cow's milk from her diet before the mother's milk is free of the substance (Jakobsson & Lindberg, 1978, 1983).
- There have been reported individual cases of other foods in the mother's diet causing reactions (eczema, proctocolitis) in the baby. Implicated foods include cow's milk, soy, eggs, wheat, and fish eaten singularly or in combination (Lucarelli et al., 2011; Pumberger, Pomberger, & Geissler, 2001).

BABY GAINING TOO FAST/TOO MUCH

After a small weight loss in the first few days after birth, exclusively breastfed infants are expected to gain about 0.5 ounce to 1 ounce or more a day.

Breastfed babies, especially exclusively breastfed babies, gain weight more rapidly in the early months (and less rapidly after 4–6 months) compared with the average baby according to standardized NCHS growth charts. As mentioned previously, standard NCHS charts show the combined growth averages of formula-fed, mixed-fed, and breastfed infants.

MANAGEMENT ISSUES

In 2010, the CDC recommended that the WHO growth curves be used to assess growth of all children under 24 months of age, a recommendation that the AAP approved in 2012. However, some breastfed babies gain much more than expected: a pound or more a week, for example, for the first 8 to 12 weeks. In the second half of the first year, they gain much less rapidly, even after starting solids. When rapidly gaining exclusively breastfed babies are compared with other exclusively breastfed babies, their growth may not seem so rapid and the fall-off of their growth rate in the second half of the first year is found to be quite typical. Growth charts for exclusively breastfed babies are now available via the WHO (Appendix Y). Those available from Health Education Associates (Appendix Y) plot exclusively breastfed infants who participated in the WHO growth study compared with babies fed a variety of ways as plotted by the NCHS.

Questions to ask:
- Is the rapidly gaining baby unhappy or unsettled after nursing?
- Does the mother have sore nipples or recurrent mastitis?
- Are the nursing sessions difficult, with the baby pulling on and off the breast?
- Does the baby have multiple large stools a day? (The stools often come out of the diaper and onto the clothes.)

If the answer is yes to two or more of these questions:
- The issue could be a condition called oversupply, where the mother is making more milk than the baby can comfortably handle. The issue is not the weight gain, and that should be made clear to

the mother. The issue is that breastfeeding is not pleasurable for mother or baby (Appendix K).

What to do about it:

- Help the mother achieve a posture where the baby is able to move his or her head freely when the flow of milk is too great or fast to handle, such as reclining or semireclining with the baby's body supported on the mother's. The mother is "down under" the baby (hence the position's title, the Australian posture), and the baby no longer has to work against the milk flow.
- Try nursing on only one breast at each feeding to allow a small amount of breast compression to tamp back the supply. A firm bra may also help. The mother must be careful not to allow too much pressure because that could foster mastitis.
- In some cases, the mother may need to use only one breast for two or more feedings in a row. This is referred to as block feeding.
- Instead of decreasing the milk supply using compression, some mothers prefer to collect the extra milk and donate to a mothers' milk bank. See Appendix Y for donation information.

In Our Experience

Oversupply is often overlooked because fear of inadequate amounts of milk pervades our consciousness.

The issue of oversupply is complicated by some of the rules that mothers are given about breastfeeding such as "nurse on each breast for 15 minutes." This mother has lots of milk, and the baby is great at transferring it. These babies may take an extraordinary amount of milk in a short time.

One can confirm that oversupply is the issue by doing before and after weights (Appendix E). Weights taken before and after nursing with a digital scale accurate to 2 grams would show rapid transfer of more than expected amounts of milk at the breast in a shorter than expected amount of time (for example, 3 ounces in 5 minutes) with the issue of oversupply. (See Appendix G for estimates of daily milk requirements.)

WORKING AND BREASTFEEDING
Mothers have worked and breastfed since the beginning of time. The difference today is that women are expected to be separated from their baby when they work outside the home. It is the separation, not the physical act of working, that complicates breastfeeding.

Working plans:
- The choice to breastfeed seems to be made independently of whether or not a woman will be working during the first year after the baby is born.
- *Expecting* to work in the first year after the baby's birth does not significantly impact whether or not a mother initiates breastfeeding.
- *The timing* of returning to work is closely linked to ending breastfeeding.
- While only 35 percent of pregnant women thought their workplace would be very supportive of breastfeeding, 52 percent of postpartum women found their workplace to be very supportive (Fein, Mandal, & Roe, 2008).
- Fein et al. (2008) reported that women used the following strategies to continue breastfeeding in the first month of work (presented from most to least prevalent):
  - Express and save milk collected to be fed to the baby later.
  - Keep the infant at work and nurse during the workday.

- ○ Neither pump nor feed during the workday.
- ○ Go to the infant to nurse during the workday.
- ○ Have the baby brought to the mother to feed during the workday.
- ○ Express and discard milk collected.
- Different strategies for combining breastfeeding and work produce significantly different breastfeeding outcomes. Strategies that included feeding directly at the breast during the day, or expressing and feeding directly during the day, were correlated with a longer breastfeeding duration (> 31.4-week and 32.4-week duration after return to work, respectively) than expressing only (26.3-week duration after return to work) and neither expressing nor feeding during the day (14.3-week duration after return to work) (Fein et al., 2008).
- Most mothers can express breastmilk for infants aged 3 to 6 months in less than an hour, distributed in about two separate sessions, in an employment environment supportive of breastfeeding (Slusser, Lange, Dickson, Hawkes, & Cohen, 2004).
- The 2010 U.S. Health Care Reform Bill included an amendment to Section 7 of the Fair Labor Standards Act requiring employers of greater than 50 employees:
  - ○ To provide "reasonable break time for an employee to express breastmilk for her nursing child for 1 year after the child's birth each time such employee has the need to express the milk."
  - ○ To provide a private place other than a bathroom.
- Company-sponsored lactation programs:
  - ○ According to Ortiz, McGilligan, and Kelly (2004), these programs "can enable mothers to provide breastmilk for their infants as long as they wish . . . even mothers who are the least likely to choose breastfeeding."

○ Services may include classes on benefits of breastfeeding, services of a lactation care provider, and private space in the workplace with equipment for pumping.

Strategies for supporting women who plan to return to work or school:
- Focus on helping new mothers to breastfeed shortly (e.g., the first week) after discharge.
- Encourage the mother to explore her options regarding the strategies identified previously. For example, can she bring her baby to work with her, at least in the short term? Or can she negotiate to work part-time at first, increasing to full-time gradually? Or work some hours weekly from her home?
- Be available as she prepares to return to work.
- Save the tips for the appropriate time, 2–3 weeks before return to work (need to know vs. nice to know).
- Make support for working mothers available in the community. Become familiar with available resources. Download the "Business Case for Breastfeeding" from the Health Resources and Services Administration Office on Women's Health (www.hrsa.gov) (Appendix Y). This package contains sample forms and resources for employers and employees.

SLEEPING THROUGH THE NIGHT
Newborn babies need to feed around the clock, whether they are breastfed or not.

- "Sleeping through the night" means a stretch of 5 to 6 hours.
- It is not realistic to expect babies to sleep more than 3 hours in a row at night until they weigh at least 10 pounds (or around 2 months of age).
- Babies will continue to awaken at night if they are not adequately fed during the daytime and evening. Although patterns vary from baby to baby,

after the early weeks, many babies "tank up" by increasing nursing frequency in the late afternoon and throughout the evening. Mothers report that this seems to be in anticipation of sleeping for a longer stretch (up to 6 hours) at night. If the mother does not meet the baby's need for frequent daytime and evening feedings, the baby may continue to awaken frequently to nurse at night.

- A baby who is not gaining well must be fed frequently at night, too. Having the baby sleeping in close proximity to the mother may help the mother respond to subtle nighttime feeding cues (AAP, 2012).

- Our motto is "daytime interventions work best for nighttime problems." Babies who have lots of naps and sleepy times during the day are less likely to sleep for longer stretches at night.

- Parents who want their babies to sleep longer at night may be attracted to "baby training" plans. This is only appropriate for babies who are gaining well and are more than 4 months old. Careful attention should be paid to the baby's reaction to baby training, including continued weight gain.

- Babies older than 6 months who had been sleeping through the night may start waking during the night again to nurse. Sometimes, this is because of teething discomfort. Teething products can be very helpful in soothing sore gums. Sometimes, this waking is because the baby is too busy during the day to get in the nursing, calories, and cuddles he or she needs. Paying more attention to daytime feedings, nursings, and cuddles may help the baby sleep longer.

SLEEPING IN CLOSE PROXIMITY TO THE MOTHER

- Babies, especially newborn babies, are safest when they sleep in close proximity to their mother. She can hear the baby and be awakened by quiet sounds and movements.

- When the baby is close to the mother, he or she can match breathing and sleep cycles to the mother's. Breastfeeding works best when the baby and mother are close.
- "Close proximity" means that the baby shares a room with his or her mother for at least the first 6 months, as this helps with breastfeeding and protects babies against sudden infant death syndrome (SIDS) (AAP Task Force on Sudden Infant Death Syndrome, 2005).
- Adult beds are not designed with infant safety in mind. Babies can die if they get trapped or wedged in the bed, or if a parent lies on them. The safest place for a baby to sleep is next to the mother's bed on his or her back.
- Side-car sleepers, bassinets, and cribs can be put next to the parents' bed. Parents who wish to sleep with the baby in their bed should carefully consider whether they could do so safely. Adult beds are not designed for babies. Couches, chairs, and recliners are not safe choices for sleeping with babies either.
- UNICEF UK (2011) provides balanced guidance to parents on issues related to safe sleep. In a companion guide to the UK UNICEF pamphlet for healthcare professionals regarding supporting safe sleep, Blair and Inch (n.d., p. 17) state:

  The over-riding message to parents in relation to bed-sharing should be:
  - *Do not sleep with your baby when you have been drinking any alcohol or taking drugs (legal or illegal) that might make you sleepy.*
  - *Do not sleep with your baby if you or anyone else in the bed is a smoker.*
  - *Do not put yourself in a position where you could doze off with your baby on a sofa/armchair.*

- If the mother is not breastfeeding, the safest place for the baby to sleep is in a safe crib or bassinet in the parents' room.

SECTION 8

Baby Feeding Problems

CONCERN: MY BABY WON'T LATCH ON

Descriptor: Baby Will Not Feed When the Mother Offers the Breast

Feeding refusal indicates that something is amiss, as it is normal for the baby to desire to suckle, even if not hungry. Feeding refusal can be:

- Continuous.
- One-sided.
- Sporadic.

Unique Identifier

Feeding refusal that is continuous.

The baby refuses to feed from the breast. Generally this refers to the baby who will not latch to the breast—although sometimes babies latch and then immediately pull off, usually crying.

Ask yourself:

- Have baby's weight gain and output been appropriate? (Appendices H, I)
- Does the baby look dehydrated, jaundiced, or otherwise malnourished? Does the baby seem alert and active, or lethargic?
- How does the mother respond to the baby's refusal?
- If the onset is sudden and refusal is continuous, what may have changed recently? For example, is the mother taking a new drug, nutritional supplement, or herb?

Watch out for:
- Presence of feeding cues prior to feeding.
- Process used to bring baby to the breast.
- Visible signs of pain for baby and mother.

What to do about it:
- Observe a feeding using the feeding observation checklist (Appendix B).
- If baby refuses to latch, ask mother to hold baby skin to skin until feeding cues are observed and baby moves toward the breast.
- Encourage the mother to bring the baby close to the breast immediately upon observation of feeding cues.
- Coach mother in trying alternate positions. Encourage her to use hand expression to release a few drops of milk to offer baby to smell and lap. If baby latches, use alternate massage/breast compression (**Figure 8-1**) to increase flow if baby becomes fidgety (Appendix D).

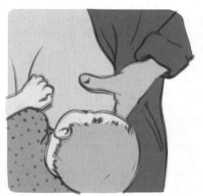

Courtesy of Healthy Children Project

Figure 8-1 Alternate massage or breast compression is a way to increase the flow of milk to the baby. The mother compresses the breast when the baby pauses.

- Coach mother on other changes to feeding process indicated by the feeding observation.
- Persist in trying to uncover the underlying reason for difficulty in coming to the breast. Babies should show desire. Not doing so raises concern.
- Schedule follow-up and ensure appropriate referrals.

Expected resolution:
- Baby and mother will be assisted with finding comfortable feeding postures and positions (Appendix C).
- If baby cannot be helped to breastfeed and the pediatric care provider has prescribed supplementation (Appendices E, F, G), encourage mother to practice skin-to-skin care as much as possible to assist baby in developing comfort being held to the breast.
- Consider at-breast supplementation if supplementation is prescribed.
- Work with mother to ensure that she is expressing milk adequately to build and/or maintain an abundant milk supply.

What else to consider:
- If observation and positioning guidance do not resolve refusal, immediate broader evaluation is required. Problems such as stuffy nose and other respiratory problems, ear or other infection, and trauma (such as fractured clavicle or torticollis) must be ruled out. Babies with neuromuscular problems, those who have experienced painful procedures to the head (for example, suctioning, intubation, or repeated examination), and those who have been forced to the breast may refuse to feed. The pediatric care provider may recommend supplementation. In this case, work with mother to maintain/build her milk supply (Appendix J) through

BABY FEEDING PROBLEMS

milk expression (Appendix M). Also consider use of an at-breast supplementer (Appendix N). Consider the mother's situation as well. If the mother is anticipating feeding pain or refusal, the baby may react negatively. If the mother's milk supply is low, or the flow is not fast, the baby who has been exposed to the bottle nipple may refuse the breast. In this case, fine-tuning the latch and positioning and using alternate breast massage/breast compression (Figure 8-1 and Appendix D) or an at-breast supplementer (Appendix N) may assist in keeping the baby at the breast. If the reason for feeding refusal is not identified via pediatric evaluation, the mother should be examined by her healthcare provider. Rarely, breast refusal has indicated abnormal process in the breast or body (e.g., cancer [Goldsmith's sign], lupus).

In Our Opinion

Feeding refusal must be taken seriously. Babies can dehydrate very quickly. It is best to err on the side of caution in these cases, particularly when the baby is a newborn.

Sometimes family or friends will suggest that the mother allow the baby to become hungry, suggesting that when the baby is hungry enough he or she will accept the breast. This is a dangerous strategy that may be detrimental to the baby's health and the parents' peace of mind.

Occasionally, feeding refusal is caused by a misunderstanding of when to feed the baby. Perhaps the mother is trying to feed the baby on a schedule, is not aware of the baby's early feeding cues, or is concerned that responding to them will "spoil" the baby. We do not believe it is possible to spoil a baby by responsive caregiving.

CONCERN: MY BABY WON'T LATCH ON

Descriptor: Baby Will Not Feed When the Mother Offers the Breast

Feeding refusal indicates that something is amiss, as it is normal for the baby to desire to suckle, even if not hungry. Feeding refusal can be:

- Continuous.
- One-sided.
- Sporadic.

Unique Identifier

Baby refuses one breast, but not the other.

Ask yourself:
- Have baby's weight gain and output been appropriate? (Appendices H, I)
- Is there something different about how the mother holds the baby on one breast versus the other?
- Is one breast or nipple substantially different from the other?
- What is the baby's body language when positioned on each breast?

Watch out for:
- Consistency of one-sided refusal. Does baby always refuse the same breast (left or right)? Or is baby refusing different breasts at different feeds? For example, the baby finishes the first breast and refuses the second because one side is sufficient at this time.

What to do about it:
- Observe a feeding using the feeding observation checklist (Appendix B).
- If baby consistently refuses the same breast:
  - Ask the mother to offer baby the preferred breast. When baby releases that breast, move baby to the other breast without shifting the baby's body position, as in **Figure 8-2**.
  - For example, consider Baby Fred who will nurse happily on the right breast, but always refuses the left. If Fred is nursing on the right breast in cradle position, ask mother to slide him over to the left, so that he is now approaching the left breast from the football position (Figure 8-2). If Fred will accept the

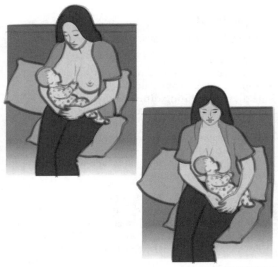

Courtesy of Healthy Children Project

Figure 8-2 The mother nurses the baby on the second breast without turning the baby over.

left breast when held in the position accepted
on the preferred breast, it may indicate some
kind of physical discomfort associated with
lying on the other side of his body (e.g., ear
infection, fractures, strains). In this case, Fred
needs pediatric evaluation.

○ If this position switch does not result in latch
on the less-favored breast, then work with
mother to try other positions. If unable to
assist baby in latching, refer mother and
baby for medical evaluation. Rarely, breast
refusal has indicated abnormal process in the
mother's breast or body (e.g., cancer, lupus)
or in the baby's body (e.g., head or brachial
plexus injury or torticollis).

• If baby prefers only one breast per feeding, but
does not always refuse the same breast:

○ Collect a prefeeding weight if possible (see
protocol in Appendix E).

○ Listen for sounds of swallowing, rhythm of
sucks to swallows, and any milk escaping from
baby's mouth during feeding.

○ In this case, it is possible that the baby is
receiving adequate milk at one breast and
cannot handle the volume from both breasts
during a feed. This is normal and reflects an
abundant milk supply. Inquire if the mother
has any discomfort associated with overfull-
ness on the unsuckled breast. If so, coach her
in learning hand expression (Appendix M)
to ease the fullness without removing much
milk (which would cause an even greater
milk supply).

○ Conduct a postfeeding weight check. Calculate
milk transfer (Appendix E). Calculate the
baby's approximate daily needs (Appendix F),
and divide that figure by the number of
reported feeds in 24 hours. How does the
amount arrived at compare with the amount
of milk transferred during this feeding?

- ○ If the transfer estimate is much lower than the estimated need, follow the protocol for poor milk supply and milk transfer (Appendices J, L).
- ○ If the transfer estimate is higher than the estimated need, follow the protocol for oversupply (Appendix K).
- ○ If the transfer estimate is roughly the same as the estimated need, schedule follow-up contact to ensure that the problem is resolving.
- ○ Note: Any single feeding does not necessarily indicate a typical milk intake. For this reason, it is helpful to observe several feedings over a period of time to get a better estimate of average transfer.
- Coach mother on other changes to feeding process indicated by the feeding observation.
- Schedule follow-up and ensure appropriate referrals.

Expected resolution:
- If the reason for one-sided refusal is identified, the problem should resolve quickly. In many cases, the mother can ensure an adequate milk supply even if the baby only suckles on one breast. However, she may need help with milk expression for comfort or to build her supply should supplementation be prescribed.

What else to consider:
- Other medical problems for mother and baby.

In Our Opinion

Differences in the rate of milk flow may describe the majority of one-sided feeding that is not restricted to the same breast at each feed. However, we must be vigilant for those cases that do not fall into this category, particularly the case where the breast refused is always the same side.

Pre- and postfeeding weight checks are a useful tool that can be overused. They should be used only when there is a genuine need to evaluate milk supply, as in the case of this presenting problem. Overuse may disempower mothers and enforce a focus on quantity of milk, rather than quality of feedings.

CONCERN: MY BABY WON'T LATCH ON

Descriptor: Baby Will Not Feed When the Mother Offers the Breast

Feeding refusal indicates that something is amiss, as it is normal for the baby to desire to suckle, even if not hungry. Feeding refusal can be:

- Continuous.
- One-sided.
- Sporadic.

Unique Identifier

Baby sporadically refuses to feed.

Ask yourself:
- Have baby's weight gain and output been appropriate?
- What factors are associated with this baby's refusal?
- What is different about those feedings in which the baby refuses the breast?

Watch out for:
- Baby's body language.
- Mother's body language.

What to do about it:

- Interview mother about conditions under which baby has refused breast (such as time of day, portion of feed during which refusal is seen [e.g., at the beginning or end of the feed, when milk flow slows or increases]; baby's hunger level, how mother decides when to feed, presence of external stressors [e.g., noise level, activity in household, before or after mother/baby separation]; and use of bottles, pacifiers, or medications for mother and baby). Probe for anything that is different about the days and times that baby refuses to feed.
- Observe a feeding using the feeding observation checklist (Appendix B).
- If baby refuses to latch during observation, ask mother to hold baby skin to skin until feeding cues are observed. Encourage mother to bring baby to the breast when feeding cues are observed.
- Coach mother in trying alternate positions. Encourage her to use hand expression (Appendix M) to release a few drops of milk to offer baby to smell and lap. If baby latches, use alternate massage/breast compression to increase flow if baby becomes fidgety (Appendix D).
- If observation and positioning guidance do not resolve refusal, comprehensive pediatric evaluation is indicated. Medical problems (e.g., stuffy nose, infection, trauma) must be ruled out. The pediatric care provider may recommend supplementation. In this case, work with mother to maintain/build her milk supply through milk expression (Appendices J, M). Use her milk preferentially to formula, and consider use of an at-breast supplementer (Appendix N).
- Coach mother on other changes to feeding process indicated by the feeding observation.
- Schedule follow-up and ensure appropriate referrals.

Expected resolution:
- When reasons for sporadic feeding refusal are identified and addressed, the problem should gradually resolve. Mothers and babies learn how to accommodate each other gradually over the early weeks of breastfeeding.

What else to consider:
- Could baby be in pain when held in certain positions? A comprehensive pediatric evaluation of baby is indicated. Babies with birth trauma, torticollis, ear infection, teething pain, and so on, may refuse feeding.
- Babies with neuromuscular problems, those who have experienced painful procedures to the head (e.g., suctioning, intubation, repeated examination), and those who have been forced to the breast may refuse to feed.
- If supplementation is prescribed:
  - Use expressed milk preferentially.
  - Encourage mother to practice skin-to-skin care as much as possible to assist baby in developing comfort being held to the breast.
  - Consider at-breast supplementation in this case.
  - Work with mother to ensure that she is expressing milk adequately to maintain an abundant milk supply.
- Consider the mother as well:
  - Could she be menstruating? (Some mothers report that babies refuse their milk, or fuss at the breast during the premenstrual and menstrual periods.)
  - Could she be using a perfumed lotion, soap, detergent, or other substance that baby dislikes?
  - Could she be taking a new or strongly flavored medication/herb/nutritional supplement periodically?

In Our Opinion

Sporadic feeding refusal typically denotes some miscoordination between mother and baby. Assisting the mother in observing and responding appropriately to the baby's cues may help overcome this problem.

CONCERN: MY BABY LATCHES ON, BUT DOESN'T STAY ATTACHED (DOESN'T SUSTAIN THE FEEDING)

This concern indicates a need for feeding observation, as the baby is unable to maintain an adequate seal at the breast, resulting in ineffective milk transfer.

Descriptor: Difficulty Keeping Baby Attached to the Breast

Unique Identifier

Baby latches to the breast but does not maintain a seal.

Ask yourself:
- Have baby's weight gain and output been appropriate?
- Does the baby appear well nourished?
- Does the baby seem appropriately interactive and interested in feeding?

Watch out for:
- Lips not sufficiently flanged out or lips rolled in.
- Mouth not open wide enough (140 to 160 degrees) to take in sufficient breast tissue.
- Potential anomalies of baby's mouth or mother's breast/nipples.
- Location of mother's hands during feeding.
- Baby's body language.

What to do about it:
- Obtain a prefeeding weight, if possible (see protocol in Appendix E).
- Observe a feeding using the feeding observation checklist (Appendix B).
- Watch closely for baby's interest in feeding. If mother is trying to feed when baby is not indicating feeding readiness, coach her on feeding cues and appropriate responses. If baby is not in a receptive state, encourage skin-to-skin contact until feeding cues are seen.
- When baby is attached to the breast and does not maintain seal, encourage mother to detach the baby and use hand expression to release a few drops of milk for the baby to smell and lap (Appendix M). Observe baby attempting to latch again. Try different positions.
- Conduct a postfeeding weight check. Calculate milk transfer. Calculate the baby's approximate daily needs (Appendix F), and divide that figure by the number of reported feeds in 24 hours. How does the amount arrived at compare with the amount of milk transferred during this feeding?
  - If the transfer estimate is much lower than the estimated need, follow the protocol for poor milk supply/transfer (Appendices J, L).
  - If the transfer estimate is higher than the estimated need, follow the protocol for oversupply (Appendix K).
  - If the transfer estimate is roughly the same as the estimated need, schedule follow-up contact to ensure that the problem is resolving.
  - Note: Any single feeding does not necessarily indicate a typical milk intake. For this reason, it is helpful to observe several feedings over a period of time to get a better estimate of average transfer.

- Coach mother on other changes to feeding process indicated by the feeding observation.
- Schedule follow-up and ensure appropriate referrals.

Expected resolution:
- When reasons for attachment difficulties are identified and addressed, the problem should gradually resolve. Mothers and babies learn how to accommodate each other gradually over the early weeks of breastfeeding.

What else to consider:
- If observation and positioning guidance do not resolve problem, refer baby to the pediatric care provider for evaluation.
- Problems such as stuffy nose, respiratory issues, tongue tie, clefts of the hard or soft palate, and neuromuscular or cardiac issues must be ruled out.
- The pediatric care provider may recommend supplementation.
- In this case, work with mother to maintain/ build her milk supply through milk expression, and encourage her to practice skin-to-skin care as much as possible to assist baby in developing comfort being held to the breast.

In Our Opinion

Babies who do not maintain a seal are telling us one of several things: Either they cannot maintain a seal due to issues such as under-nourishment, attachment problem, or intraoral structural or neuromuscular problem, or they do not want to maintain a seal (perhaps because the rate of milk flow is too fast or because the nipple extends too far into their mouth, triggering the gag reflex).

CONCERN: MY BABY IS NOT COMFORTABLE AT THE BREAST

Descriptor: Baby Expresses Distress Related to Feeding

Babies may express discomfort at the breast in many ways. These can include:

- Fretting at the breast.
- Crying at the breast.

Unique Identifier

Baby frets at the breast.

This baby is expressing distress during feedings through sounds and body language. Mothers may describe this behavior as fussing, or fretting, at the breast or as the baby not wanting to stay at the breast. The physical behaviors of the baby may include pushing away from the breast, batting at the breast, and so on.

Ask yourself:

- Is baby exhibiting expected familiarization behaviors that are being interpreted as discomfort? For example, the newborn often attaches several times with a small degree of mouth opening before settling into a deeper latch with rhythmic suckling.
- Have baby's weight gain and output been appropriate?
- Does mother demonstrate an understanding of baby's feeding cues and respond appropriately?
- Could baby be having difficulty breathing?
- Could baby be having trouble coordinating sucking, swallowing, and breathing?
- Could baby be in pain?
- Could mother be in pain?

BABY FEEDING PROBLEMS

Watch out for:
- Changes in baby's body position or mother's hand position during feeding.
- Changes in baby's lip and facial skin color during a feeding (e.g., becoming pale, gray, or blue). These changes may indicate an undiagnosed physical problem for baby. Comprehensive pediatric evaluation is urgently required before attempting another oral feeding.
- Fretting or pulling away that appears to be necessary for baby to breathe. In these cases, consider a swallowing, coordination, or respiratory problem. Comprehensive pediatric evaluation is urgently required before attempting another oral feeding.

What to do about it:
- Observe a feeding using the feeding observation checklist (Appendix B).
- Watch closely for baby's interest in feeding. If mother is trying to feed when baby is not indicating feeding readiness, coach her on feeding cues and appropriate responses. If baby is not in a receptive state, encourage skin-to-skin contact, allowing baby to self-attach or begin collaborative feeding when feeding cues are seen.
- When attached to the breast, if baby begins to fret, encourage mother to detach the baby and hold him or her skin to skin until feeding cues are seen again. Then watch the process closely to see if there is a difference in the baby's or mother's body position before and after the fretting begins.
- If fretting continues, try different positions.
- Ask the mother to use alternate massage/breast compression (Appendix D) to change the rate of flow of the milk. Observe for sucking and swallowing. Does baby begin to fret when the milk is flowing rapidly or slowly? (Listen to the suck-to-swallow ratio to answer this question.

Nutritive flow is thought to occur at one or two sucks per swallow.)
- Coach mother on other changes to feeding process indicated by the feeding observation.
- Schedule follow-up and/or ensure appropriate referrals.

Expected resolution:
- The behavior should resolve when the problem is identified and appropriately addressed. If the change requires a way of holding baby, it may take some time for the mother/baby to finesse the new position.
- Encourage mother to return for a follow-up observation to fine-tune the positioning.

What else to consider:
- If the problem cannot be resolved, the baby requires a comprehensive pediatric evaluation. In some cases, stuffy nose, as well as more serious problems such as submucosal clefts and other anomalies, have been associated with this behavior.

In Our Opinion

Hungry babies often exhibit this fretting behavior. Mothers may misread the baby's behavior of batting at the breast as anger; however, it may also reflect the baby's kneading behavior at the breast, which has been associated with increased oxytocin and, thus, enhanced milk flow. Similarly, the baby "pulling away" may be the baby pushing back against something that is restricting his or her ability to get the widest mouth opening, which the breastfed baby comes to associate with the greatest milk flow rate. One of the most helpful acts of the supportive lactation care provider may be helping the mother to read the baby's body language correctly.

CONCERN: MY BABY IS NOT COMFORTABLE AT THE BREAST

Descriptor: Baby Expresses Distress Related to Feeding

Babies may express discomfort at the breast in many ways. These can include:

- Fretting at the breast.
- Crying at the breast.

Unique Identifier

Baby cries at the breast.

The baby is expressing distress during the feeding by pulling away and crying. This may happen before or during feeding.

Ask yourself:
- Have the baby's weight gain and output been appropriate?
- Could the baby be in pain?
- Could the mother be misreading the baby's feeding cues?
- Could the mother be delaying feedings?

Watch out for:
- Feeding cues and mother's response.
- Position of baby and mother before and after the crying starts.

What to do about it:
- Observe a feeding using the feeding observation checklist (Appendix B).
- Watch closely for baby's interest in feeding. If mother is trying to feed when baby is not indicating feeding readiness, coach her on feeding cues and appropriate responses. If baby is not in a receptive state, encourage skin-to-skin contact, allowing the baby to self-attach or

begin collaborative feeding when feeding cues are seen.

- If baby begins to cry when attached to the breast, encourage mother to detach the baby and hold him or her skin to skin, allowing the baby to self-attach or begin collaborative feeding when feeding cues are seen. Then watch the process closely to see if there is a difference in the baby's or mother's body position before and after the fretting begins. Look for restriction of the baby's head, position of the baby's arms and legs, and so on.
- If crying continues, try different positions.
- Ask the mother to use alternate massage/breast compression (Appendix D) to change the rate of flow of the milk. Observe for sucking and swallowing. Does baby begin to cry when the milk is flowing rapidly or when it is not flowing?
- Coach mother on other changes to feeding process indicated by the feeding observation.
- Schedule follow-up and ensure appropriate referrals.

Expected resolution:
- The behavior should resolve when the problem is identified and appropriately addressed. If the change requires a different way of holding baby, it may take some time for the mother/baby to finesse the new position.
- Encourage mother to return for a follow-up observation to fine-tune the positioning.

What else to consider:
- If the problem cannot be resolved, a comprehensive pediatric evaluation is indicated. Problems such as stuffy nose, teething pain, injuries such as fractured clavicle or brachial plexus injury, and other anomalies have been associated with this behavior.

In Our Opinion

It is unfortunate that American culture equates crying with hunger. The baby who is crying is telling us that something is wrong.

CONCERN: I'M WORRIED ABOUT MY MILK SUPPLY (FIGURE 8-3)

Descriptor: Concern about Adequacy of Milk Supply

Many mothers are concerned that they will not produce an adequate amount of milk. Their friends and family may support this concern. Among the factors that may increase this concern are the following:

- *Baby has not gained an adequate amount of weight.*
- Baby falls asleep after just a few minutes of feeding.
- Baby seems unsatisfied after feedings.
- Breasts feel "empty."
- Expressed milk volume is less than expected.

Unique Identifier

Poor weight gain in the baby is reported.

Baby's weight gain is thought to be problematic or has been measured and found inadequate.

Ask yourself:
- Has the baby's pediatric care provider identified a problem with the baby's weight gain pattern?
- Has baby's output been appropriate? (Appendix I)
- Does baby appear dehydrated? Jaundiced? Malnourished?
- Is baby's behavior appropriately interactive?

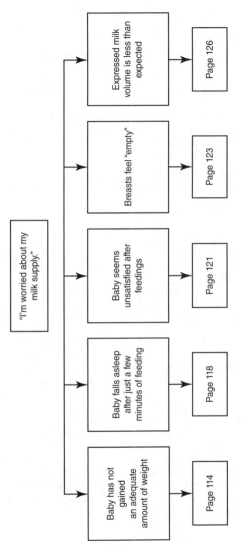

Figure 8-3 I'm worried about my milk supply.

"I'm worried about my milk supply."

Baby has not gained an adequate amount of weight	Baby falls asleep after just a few minutes of feeding	Baby seems unsatisfied after feedings	Breasts feel "empty"	Expressed milk volume is less than expected
Page 114	Page 118	Page 121	Page 123	Page 126

Watch out for:
- Mother's knowledge of and response to baby's cues.
- Possibility of inaccuracy of measurements (e.g., weights taken on different or inaccurate scale[s]).
- Use of an inappropriate growth chart to track the growth of exclusively breastfed babies, especially after 4–6 months. The WHO growth curve should be used for all babies under 24 months.

What to do about it:
- Obtain a prefeeding weight if possible (see protocol in Appendix E).
- Observe a feeding using the feeding observation checklist (Appendix B).
- Observe baby's approach to the breast. Does baby exhibit interest in feeding? Does baby seem to be conserving energy, or is he or she actively feeding?
- When baby is attached to the breast, observe for sucking and swallowing.
- If baby stops suckling and appears to go to sleep, ask the mother to use alternate massage/breast compression (Appendix D) to change the rate of flow of the milk. Observe for sucking and swallowing. Does baby get more wakeful and suckle more actively? Or does baby break suction?
- Conduct a postfeeding weight check. Calculate milk transfer. Calculate the baby's approximate daily needs (Appendix F), and divide that figure by the amount of reported feeds in 24 hours. How does the amount arrived at compare with the amount of milk transferred during this feeding?
  - If the transfer estimate is much lower than the estimated need, follow the protocol for poor milk supply/transfer (Appendices J, L). The pediatric care provider should determine the need for supplementation.

○ Note: Any one feeding does not necessarily indicate a typical milk intake. For this reason, it is helpful to observe several feedings over a period of time to get a better estimate of average transfer.

- Coach mother on other changes to feeding process indicated by the feeding observation.
- Schedule follow-up and ensure appropriate referrals.

Expected resolution:

- When a weight gain problem is confirmed, intensive pediatric follow-up and breastfeeding assessment and education are indicated. In most cases, milk supply can be increased, and milk transfer can be improved.
- If a milk supply and/or transfer problem is not confirmed, additional follow-up is indicated to ensure appropriate growth.

What else to consider:

- The pediatric care provider may prescribe supplementation. In this case, work with mother to maintain/build her milk supply through milk expression (Appendices J, M). Use expressed milk preferentially as a supplement and consider use of an at-breast supplementer (Appendix N) to deliver supplement or expressed milk.
- If a milk supply/transfer problem is confirmed, but not explained by pediatric evaluation, a comprehensive maternal medical evaluation is indicated. Occasionally, medical issues such as endocrine insufficiency, polycystic ovarian syndrome, medications, superimposed pregnancy, and other conditions have been associated with milk production problems.

In Our Opinion

It is essential to explore this concern fully with mothers. Too many mothers are told not to worry about their milk supply or to go to bed and nurse their babies to increase their milk supply. Any concern raised by a mother deserves our full exploration and examination. No matter how common a concern among women, we have no way of knowing when we are dealing with a situation that is far from either common or normal. There is a traditional saying that mothers know when something is wrong; strive to honor women's knowledge by fully exploring their concerns, no matter how common.

CONCERN: I'M WORRIED ABOUT MY MILK SUPPLY

Descriptor: Concern about Adequacy of Milk Supply

Many mothers are concerned that they will not produce an adequate amount of milk. Their friends and family may support this concern. Among the factors that may increase this concern are the following:

- Baby has not gained an adequate amount of weight.
- *Baby falls asleep after just a few minutes of feeding.*
- Baby seems unsatisfied after feedings.
- Breasts feel "empty."
- Expressed milk volume is less than expected.

Unique Identifier

Baby falls asleep after just a few minutes of feeding.

Mothers may have been told that feeding baby will take a certain amount of time. They may be concerned about their milk supply when their baby nurses for a shorter time and then falls asleep.

Ask yourself:
- Have baby's weight gain and output been appropriate?
- Does baby appear dehydrated? Jaundiced? Malnourished?
- Is baby's behavior appropriately interactive?

Watch out for:
- Mother's knowledge of and response to baby's cues.
- Misreading of quiet-alert stage with eyes closed as "sleeping" (active feeding can occur during baby states that look inactive).

What to do about it:
- Obtain a prefeeding weight if possible (see protocol in Appendix E).
- Observe a feeding using the feeding observation checklist (Appendix B).
- Watch closely for baby's interest in feeding. If mother is trying to feed when baby is not indicating feeding readiness, coach her on feeding cues and appropriate responses. If baby is not in a receptive state, encourage skin-to-skin contact until feeding cues are seen.
- When baby is attached to the breast, observe for sucking and swallowing.
- If baby stops suckling and appears to go to sleep, ask the mother to use alternate massage (Appendix D) to change the rate of flow of the milk. Observe for sucking and swallowing. Does baby get more wakeful and suckle more actively? Or does baby break suction?
- Conduct a postfeeding weight check. Calculate milk transfer. Calculate the baby's approximate daily needs (Appendix F), and divide that figure

by the number of reported feeds in 24 hours.
How does the amount arrived at compare with the
amount of milk transferred during this feeding?

○ If the transfer estimate is much lower than the
estimated need, follow the protocol for poor
milk supply/transfer (Appendices J, L).

○ If the transfer estimate is higher than the
estimated need, follow the protocol for oversupply (Appendix K).

○ If the transfer estimate is roughly the same as
the estimated need, schedule follow-up contact
to ensure that the problem is resolving.

○ Note: Any one feeding does not necessarily
indicate a typical milk intake. For this reason,
it is helpful to observe several feedings over
a period of time to get a better estimate of
average transfer.

• Coach mother on other changes to feeding
process indicated by the feeding observation.

• Schedule follow-up and ensure appropriate
referrals.

Expected resolution:

• When reasons for sleepiness are identified and
addressed, the problem should gradually resolve.
Mothers and babies grow to learn how to accommodate each other gradually over the early weeks
of breastfeeding.

What else to consider:

• If baby is a newborn, consider near-term or
prematurity, labor analgesia/anesthesia, infection, and hypoglycemia as possible contributing
factors.

• Ensure comprehensive pediatric evaluation.

In Our Opinion

There is no "right" amount of time for a feeding to last. However, mother's concerns about

feedings that are too short (or too long) always warrant a feeding evaluation. Although most newborn babies have longer feeds, as they learn how to feed effectively, experienced babies may be able to transfer significant volumes of milk in a very short amount of time (as little as 5 minutes in some cases).

CONCERN: I'M WORRIED ABOUT MY MILK SUPPLY

Descriptor: Concern about Adequacy of Milk Supply

Many mothers are concerned that they will not produce an adequate amount of milk. Their friends and family may support this concern. Among the factors that may increase this concern are the following:

- Baby has not gained an adequate amount of weight.
- Baby falls asleep after just a few minutes of feeding.
- *Baby seems unsatisfied after feedings.*
- Breasts feel "empty."
- Expressed milk volume is less than expected.

Unique Identifier

After breastfeeding, the baby is unsettled and fretful.

Ask yourself:
- Have baby's weight gain and output been appropriate?
- Does baby appear dehydrated? Jaundiced? Malnourished?
- Is baby's behavior appropriately interactive?
- Does baby only get attention and skin contact during feedings?

Watch out for:
- Mother's knowledge of and response to baby's cues.

What to do about it:
- Obtain a prefeeding weight if possible (see protocol in Appendix E).
- Observe a feeding using the feeding observation checklist (Appendix B).
- Watch closely for baby's interest in feeding. If mother is trying to feed when baby is not indicating feeding readiness, coach her on feeding cues and appropriate responses. If baby is not in a receptive state, encourage skin-to-skin contact, allowing the baby to self-attach or begin collaborative feeding when feeding cues are seen.
- When baby is attached to the breast, observe for sucking and swallowing.
- Conduct a postfeeding weight check. Calculate milk transfer. Calculate the baby's approximate daily needs (Appendix F), and divide that figure by the amount of reported feeds in 24 hours. How does the amount arrived at compare with the amount of milk transferred during this feeding?
  - If the transfer estimate is much lower than the estimated need, follow the protocol for poor milk supply/transfer (Appendices J, L).
  - If the transfer estimate is higher than the estimated need, follow the protocol for oversupply (Appendix K).
  - If the transfer estimate is roughly the same as the estimated need, schedule follow-up contact to ensure that the problem is resolving.
  - Note: Any one feeding does not necessarily indicate a typical milk intake. For this reason, it is helpful to observe several feedings over a period of time to get a better estimate of average transfer.
- Coach mother on other changes to feeding process indicated by the feeding observation.
- Schedule follow-up and/or ensure appropriate referrals.

Expected resolution:
• When baby is in a receptive feeding state and able to transfer adequate milk, this problem should resolve. Encourage parents to provide lots of non-feeding snuggling and interaction with baby to meet baby's contact needs.

What else to consider:
• Comprehensive pediatric evaluation. Teething, ear infections, and other issues can drive the baby to seek the breast for comfort.

In Our Opinion

It is thought that some babies, if not offered cuddles and attention between feedings, may demand frequent feeds to meet their need for comforting touch. We cannot say enough about the importance of cuddling and skin contact to calm, soothe, and nurture babies and their parents.

Concern: I'm Worried About My Milk Supply

Descriptor: Concern about Adequacy of Milk Supply

Many mothers are concerned that they will not produce an adequate amount of milk. Their friends and family may support this concern. Among the factors that may increase this concern are the following:

• Baby has not gained an adequate amount of weight.
• Baby falls asleep after just a few minutes of feeding.
• Baby seems unsatisfied after feedings.
• *Breasts feel "empty."*
• Expressed milk volume is less than expected.

Unique Identifier

Mother reports that her breasts feel empty.

Ask yourself:
- Could the mother be experiencing the normal breast changes of the first month of breastfeeding?
- Could the mother be experiencing breast changes consistent with long-term nursing (the change of milk production from hormonally regulated to production on demand)?
- Have baby's weight gain and output been appropriate?
- Does baby appear dehydrated? Jaundiced? Malnourished?

What to do about it:
- If there are no indications of a milk supply and/or intake problem, discuss normal breast changes with mother. Observe a feeding and evaluate using the feeding observation checklist (Appendix B).
- If the history of the problem and baby's weight gain indicate a possible milk supply or intake problem, take the following steps:
  - Obtain a prefeeding weight if possible (see protocol in Appendix E).
  - Observe a feeding using the feeding observation checklist (Appendix B).
  - Conduct a postfeeding weight check. Calculate milk transfer. Calculate the baby's approximate daily needs (Appendix F), and divide that figure by the amount of reported feeds in 24 hours. How does the amount arrived at compare with the amount of milk transferred during this feeding?
  - If the transfer estimate is much lower than the estimated need, follow the protocol for poor milk supply/transfer (Appendices J, L).

- ○ If the transfer estimate is higher than the estimated need, follow the protocol for oversupply (Appendix K).
- ○ If the transfer estimate is roughly the same as the estimated need, schedule follow-up contact to ensure that the problem is resolving.
- ○ Note: Any one feeding does not necessarily indicate a typical milk intake. For this reason, it is helpful to observe several feedings over a period of time to get a better estimate of average transfer.
- Coach mother on other changes to feeding process indicated by the feeding observation.
- Schedule follow-up and ensure appropriate referrals.

Expected resolution:
- When concern about milk supply is not confirmed by problems with the baby's growth, the mother's fears may diminish with empathetic counseling.
- When potential milk supply/intake problems are confirmed by poor growth in the baby, resolution varies with the nature of the underlying problem. In rare cases, it may not be possible for mothers to produce a full milk supply. Frequent follow-up is indicated.

What else to consider:
- Comprehensive pediatric evaluation. Teething, ear infections, and other issues can drive the baby to seek the breast for comfort.
- Maternal physical evaluation, including hormonal levels. Physical problems such as retained placental fragments, thyroid and other hormone problems, polycystic ovarian syndrome, and history of breast surgery and trauma have been associated with inadequate milk production.

BABY FEEDING PROBLEMS

In Our Opinion

Many women experience persistent concern about milk supply. Acknowledging, normalizing, and exploring this concern is indicated. Her concern should be taken seriously, regardless of the baby's growth.

CONCERN: I'M WORRIED ABOUT MY MILK SUPPLY

Descriptor: Concern about Adequacy of Milk Supply

Many mothers are concerned that they will not produce an adequate amount of milk. Their friends and family may support this concern. Among the factors that may increase this concern are the following:

- Baby has not gained an adequate amount of weight.
- Baby falls asleep after just a few minutes of feeding.
- Baby seems unsatisfied after feedings.
- Breasts feel "empty."
- *Expressed milk volume is less than expected.*

Unique Identifier

Mother reports a small quantity of expressed milk.

Ask yourself:
- How new is the mother to milk expression?
- What methods is she using to collect her milk?
- Have baby's weight gain and output been appropriate?
- Is this a new phenomenon?

What to do about it:
- If there are no indications of a milk supply and/or intake problem:
  - Acknowledge this common experience: Tell mother that most women express only a few droplets of milk initially as they become accustomed to milk expression.
  - If this is a change (gradual or a sudden drop in milk expression volume), explore changes or additions to mother's routines (e.g., mother taking new medications, nutritional supplements, or herbs; decreased number of feedings or expressions; changes to any pumping equipment; onset of menstruation; onset of new pregnancy, etc.).
  - Coach mother on milk expression techniques (Appendix M). Encourage nipple stimulation and massage prior to expression and the use of guided imagery and other tools that may enhance milk flow.
  - If the mother is using a breast pump, check the pump for missing parts or assembly problems. Ask the manufacturer how to check the pressure generated by the pump. Observe her using the pump and check for appropriate technique and good fit of the pump.
  - If the mother is only using a breast pump, encourage her to consider adding hand expression (Flaherman et al., 2011; Morton et al., 2009) (Appendix M).
  - Ask her to consider expressing the unsuckled breast while nursing baby (the oxytocin produced by the baby may increase expression yield), or to combine hand expression with pumping.
  - Encourage her to track her expression volume over time, expecting a gradual increase.

BABY FEEDING PROBLEMS

- If the history of the problem and baby's weight gain indicate a possible milk supply or intake problem, undertake a feeding observation (Appendix B).
  - Coach mother on other changes to feeding process indicated by the feeding observation.
- Schedule follow-up and ensure appropriate referrals.

Expected resolution:
- Most women become more adept at milk expression with practice.
- In cases where a milk supply problem is confirmed, milk expression can assist in stimulating milk production. Milk expressed may be used to supplement the baby if supplementation is prescribed.

What else to consider:
- If milk cannot be expressed from the breast or colostrum is expressed beyond the first 4 days of life, a comprehensive maternal medical evaluation is indicated. Problems such as retained placental fragments and history of breast surgery have been associated with the phenomenon of not moving on to adequate production of milk as expected.

In Our Opinion

It seems that many women imagine that they will express a full bottle of milk on their very first attempt. This is a very rare experience. The woman must learn to trick her body into "letting down" to her hand or the pump. (What pump is as adorable as her baby?) It takes time for most women to become adept at expressing milk.

Hand expression is a vastly underrated skill. All women should learn this valuable skill during their hospital stay.

CONCERN: MY BABY WON'T TAKE A BOTTLE/CUP

Descriptor: Baby Refuses to Drink from a Bottle or Cup

Unique Identifier

Baby refuses alternate feeding methods.

Ask yourself:
- Who has attempted to feed this baby? Mother? Father? Daycare provider? Other family member?
- What has been offered to the baby? Expressed milk? Formula? Other beverages?
- Where has feeding been attempted (in the presence or absence of the nursing mother)?
- When has feeding been attempted? Explore cue state of baby, separation from mother, and so on.
- Why has alternate feeding been attempted (e.g., separation due to return to work/school, occasional relief feeding)?
- How has fluid been offered (what devices have been used—bottles, teats, cups, spoons, etc.)?

Watch out for:
- Cue state of baby at time of attempted feeding.
- Parental response to cue state of baby.
- Manner in which baby is held for feeding.

What to do about it:
- Interview mother about attempts that have been made to feed baby with a bottle or cup. Ask the questions from the preceding "Ask yourself" section.

- Observe an attempted feeding. Encourage bottle/cup or other method to be offered when baby is in a quiet/alert stage and not exhibiting signs of overt hunger.
- Encourage that feeding be preceded by some gentle, pleasurable interaction with the individual who will feed the baby. (Note: It is often easier for babies to accept an alternate feeding device from someone other than their nursing mother. Babies may be confused by the sensory cues they receive when in their mother's presence and may not be as able to focus on learning a new way of feeding when in close proximity to her. Some babies even refuse to accept an alternate feeding method when they can see, hear, smell, or otherwise sense their mother's presence in the home.)
- Encourage the person who is feeding the baby to begin by gently massaging around baby's lips with clean fingers. The purpose of this action is to draw baby's attention to the mouth in a pleasurable way.
- Once baby shows some interest in the massage (e.g., turning head toward the stimulus, opening mouth), the bottle or cup should be raised to baby's lips.
  - If using a bottle, try one with a large dome around the nipple, as this can be used to simulate the "wide-open" mouth position of the baby feeding at the breast.
  - If using a cup, use appropriate cup-feeding technique (Appendix N). Coach the parents to raise the cup just so that fluid touches the baby's mouth, rather than pouring fluid into the baby's mouth.
- Let the baby pace the feeding. The baby should be allowed to rest as needed during the feed and allowed to stop when ready. Baby's eyes may be closed during part or all of the feeding.

Expected resolution:
- It may take time for the baby to learn to accept a new feeding method. Babies typically come to accept alternate feeding devices after some exposure to them.

What else to consider:
- Consider other methods of supplementation. The baby who will not accept a bottle may be happy with cup feeding. Other babies prefer fluid from the spoon or sip-type cup. If the alternate feeding device is being used to supplement the baby who is not receiving enough milk at the breast, and the mother is able to feed at the breast, consider at-breast supplementation (Appendix N).
- Comprehensive pediatric evaluation is needed if refusal is strong or consistent. Rarely, a suck/swallow or other intraoral problem has been discovered in these cases.

In Our Opinion

It is never appropriate to support the common belief that babies will learn to feed in a different manner when they are hungry enough. Although those who espouse this belief do so in an attempt to reassure the parents, it may lead to the unfortunate practice of "starving the baby out." Very hungry babies have less energy and patience for learning new feeding methods. Babies may also come to distrust those around them, as caregivers are not responding to the baby's need for food, a primal need that should never be ignored.

There are pros and cons to all alternate feeding devices. Be prepared to aid parents in choosing a method that protects milk production and suits their baby's abilities and their own skills and situation.

CONCERN: MY BABY WON'T SLEEP THROUGH THE NIGHT

Descriptor: Baby's Sleep Pattern Does Not Match Parental Expectations

Unique Identifier

Parental expectation of baby's nighttime sleep pattern is not being met.

Ask yourself:
• How old is the baby?
• How long has this problem existed?
• What does "sleeping through the night" mean to this family?
• How many hours is baby sleeping in a stretch at night? During the day?
• When does baby go down to sleep for the night?
• When does baby awaken mother for feedings?
• Have baby's weight gain and output been appropriate?

Watch out for:
• Unreasonable expectations about infant sleep. The longest stretch of sleep that can be expected in a breastfed baby after the newborn period is one 5- to 6-hour stretch per 24 hours. If the baby sleeps for 5 to 6 hours during the day, he or she probably will not be able to repeat a sleep of that length at night and gain adequate weight.
• Some babies wake frequently at night when they do not have adequate access to human milk during the day. This can be due to maternal distraction (e.g., a mother with many demands on her time may not notice early feeding cues, babies who spend a lot of time in the car may be lulled to sleep more often during the day) or infant distraction (e.g., around 4 to 6 months, many babies become distracted during the day by other activities, such as creeping and crawling,

and feed less often). Either maternal or infant distraction can lead to more night feeding.

What to do about it:
- Explore the baby's sleep pattern with the mother.
- Compare the baby's daily sleep pattern with age-appropriate expectations (see preceding section).
- Identify whether there is a problem with the baby's growth or other suggestions that the baby may be feeding at night to make up for lost daytime feeding opportunities.
- If day/night imbalance problems are discovered, encourage the family to work on changing the daytime patterns first. For example, if the baby is sleeping 5 to 6 hours during the day, encourage the caregiver to observe the sleeping baby and pick baby up when light sleep stage (marked by rapid eye movement under the lids) is seen. This baby can be easily moved to an awake state and can be gently offered a feeding while his or her eyes are still closed.

Expected resolution:
- Feeding the baby more often during the daytime will lead to less awakening at night.

What else to consider:
- Comprehensive pediatric evaluation. Babies who are in pain may awaken more often and seek food for comfort. Pain can result from teething, ear infection, and other problems.

In Our Opinion

A discrepancy between parental sleep expectations and reality is one of the most difficult problems for the sleep-deprived family to solve. Encourage families to adopt a proximate sleep environment—meaning that the baby sleeps in close proximity to the parents—in the same room, in a safe sleep environment. Ideally, in the first weeks mothers should sleep during the day when their babies sleep. More information about safe sleep can be found in Section 7.

CONCERN: MY BABY WON'T STOP CRYING
Descriptor: Baby Is Inconsolable
Unique Identifier
Parents are unable to soothe their crying baby.

Ask yourself:
- How long has this problem existed?
- What preceded the crying?
- What methods have been used to attempt to calm the baby?

Watch out for:
- The truly inconsolable baby needs urgent medical evaluation.
- Baby's cue state.
- Parental response to baby's cue state.
- Visible symptoms of pain or distress.

What to do about it:
- Encourage skin-to-skin contact to calm baby. Calm the environment: Consider sound, light, motion, and so on.
- Suggest other comfort techniques as needed, such as massage, rocking, singing, and bathing.
- Encourage mother to offer the breast when baby demonstrates feeding cues.

What else to consider:
- If these techniques do not calm the baby's crying, or any of the pediatric warning signs (Appendix Z) are seen, the baby needs emergent care.

- The family of the baby who cries repeatedly needs support. Family members may need some "time-out" opportunities to care for themselves.

See also:
- Colic.

In Our Opinion

Crying babies deserve comfort. Crying does not exercise the lungs or serve any helpful purpose for the baby. In the young or ill baby, excessive crying can be detrimental to growth, as it burns calories.

CONCERN: MY BABY WON'T WAKE UP ENOUGH TO NURSE WELL

Descriptor: Baby Acts Sleepy and Disinterested in Breastfeeding

Unique Identifier

Sleepy baby.

Ask yourself:
- How old is the baby?
- When did the problem begin?
- Have baby's weight gain and output been appropriate?
- Do parents understand and respond to feeding cues?

Watch out for:
- True inability to awaken needs emergent medical evaluation.
- Breathing problems in baby require urgent medical evaluation.
- Inadequate urinations and/or stooling in baby (calorically deprived babies seem sleepy) require urgent medical evaluation.

BABY FEEDING PROBLEMS

- Diagnosed congenital anomalies and neurologic problems can result in arousal difficulties.

What to do about it:
- Encourage mother to observe baby sleeping and to pick baby up and bring him or her to the breast when signs of light sleep are seen (e.g., eyes moving under the lids, small movements of the body, changes in facial expression, sounds).
- Hold the baby skin to skin between feedings to improve motor and state organization.
- Explore the baby's sleep environment. When babies are very warmly dressed/wrapped, they may sleep longer. Swaddled babies may not rouse themselves as easily when transitioning from deep to light sleep.
- Take a feeding history. Determine if an adequate number of effective feedings is occurring in a 24-hour time period (10 to 12 feeds per 24 hours for a newborn).
- Ensure comprehensive pediatric evaluation for the indication of recurring pattern of low frequency of feed or difficulty rousing baby from deep sleep.

Expected resolution:
- Mother and baby will learn to regulate sleep/ wake and feeding patterns when mother becomes adept at reading baby's language.
- In the newborn, recovery from birth, as well as exposure to labor and delivery pain medication administered to the mother and/or analgesia/ anesthesia given directly to the baby for painful procedures, may result in transient changes to the normal sleep/wake cycle.

What else to consider:
- Could the baby be marginally nourished, jaundiced, or dealing with infection or other condition? Ensure comprehensive pediatric

evaluation of weight gain problems, development, output, and sleep patterns.
- Explore daytime patterns in the baby's environment. Might there be too much environmental stimulation, such as sound or light, causing baby to shut down?

See also:
- Jaundice.

In Our Opinion

A baby's ability to rouse easily from deep sleep can be lifesaving in the event of apnea. Parents are justified in their concern about babies who have long periods of deep sleep.

CONCERN: MY BABY HAS COLIC

Descriptor: Uncomfortable Baby with Symptoms of Colic

Colic was described by Wessel and colleagues (1954) as a condition of infancy described by the classic rule of 3: bouts of high-pitched crying lasting more than 3 hours/day, for more than 3 days/week, and for more than 3 weeks in a well-nourished, otherwise healthy baby. Colic typically starts after 2 weeks of age and resolves by 4 months.

Unique Identifier

Prolonged and specific crying in a breastfed baby.

Ask yourself:
- What was the baby's age at onset?
- When did the problem begin?
- Who has diagnosed this problem as colic? The pediatric care provider? The mother?

Watch out for:
• When the symptoms occur.

What to do about it:
• Explore the history of the problem.
• Observe a feeding using the feeding observation checklist (Appendix B), looking for any problems that may increase baby's gastric discomfort (e.g., baby crying before or during feeds may introduce extra air into the digestive system; a large milk supply or fast rate of flow of milk may increase baby's gastric discomfort).
• Teach parents soothing methods: singing to baby, rocking, walking, skin-to-skin comfort, infant massage, and so on.
• Encourage parents to take turns having "time-out," if needed, from the distraught child.

Expected resolution:
• Colic symptoms typically begin after 2 weeks of age and resolve by 4 months. Changing the mother's diet may alleviate colic in some cases. The major causes of colic are unexplained but thought to be related to the development of the gastrointestinal and nervous systems.

What else to consider:
• Specialized gastrointestinal evaluation.
• A trial of removing dairy foods (especially liquid milk) from mother's diet may be conducted for 10 to 14 days to determine if colic symptoms decrease. If symptoms do not change, the mother should resume her normal diet.

See also:
• Crying.

In Our Opinion

Most babies have gastric discomfort. This does not necessarily indicate colic. Mothers will often restrict their diet severely, often without positive effect on the baby's symptoms. This may be completely unnecessary, as only a portion of colic cases can be alleviated by changes to baby's or mother's diet. If a dietary trial does not alleviate symptoms, encourage the mother to resume her normal diet and focus on helping the family learn healthy coping skills for responding to the baby's discomfort.

CONCERN: MY BABY HAS JAUNDICE

Descriptor: Visible Yellow Coloration of the Baby's Skin and Possibly the Whites of the Baby's Eyes

Unique Identifier

Jaundice in the breastfed baby.

Ask yourself:
- When was jaundice diagnosed?
- Who diagnosed it?
- What was the baby's age at onset?
- What was the gestational age of the baby at birth?

Watch out for:
- Signs of dehydration (e.g., sunken fontanelles, decreased urination, "brick dust" urine, decreased stooling).

What to do about it:
- Confer with the pediatric care provider about feeding plan.
- Observe a feeding, using the feeding observation checklist (Appendix B).
- Assess milk transfer using pre- and postfeeding weight checks (Appendix E).
- Work with mother to improve milk supply if needed.

BABY FEEDING PROBLEMS

- Ensure comprehensive pediatric evaluation as needed.
- If the mother has any condition that might limit milk production, ensure that the pediatric clinician is apprised.

Expected resolution:
- Babies with jaundice may be somewhat lethargic. Milk expression (Appendix M) and alternate massage (Appendix D) during feedings may help to increase the milk supply and intake.
- Once jaundice resolves, the baby's ability to feed should normalize.

What else to consider:
- Avoid use of a bottle or other feeding device with a firm teat. At-breast supplementation is ideal in this situation. If baby is supplemented away from the breast, consider supplementation via cup.

See also:
- Sleepy baby.

In Our Opinion

Slight jaundice in a full-term, healthy, breastfed baby appears to be normal. According to the American Academy of Pediatrics (AAP, 2004, p. 297):

In every infant, we recommend that clinicians:

1. *Promote and support successful breastfeeding.*
2. *Perform a systematic assessment before discharge for the risk of severe hyperbilirubinemia.*
3. *Provide early and focused follow-up based on the risk assessment, and when indicated, treat newborns with phototherapy or exchange transfusion to prevent the development of severe hyperbilirubinemia and, possibly, bilirubin encephalopathy (kernicterus).*

However, high levels of bilirubin may indicate that there were disturbances to early feeding and contact with mother, or an underlying medical condition, such as G6PD, glucose-6-phosphate-dehydrogenase deficiency.

Due to the fear of kernicterus, jaundice must be appropriately identified and treated. Human milk is the ideal food for all babies, including those with jaundice.

CONCERN: MY BABY HAS HYPOGLYCEMIA

Descriptor: Hypoglycemia

Hypoglycemia is a condition in which the amount of blood glucose (sugar) in the blood is lower than normal.

Unique Identifier

Hypoglycemia in the breastfed infant.

Ask yourself:
- Is this baby at higher risk for hypoglycemia (AAP Committee on Fetus and Newborn, 2011)?
  - $> 4,000$ g or $< 2,500$ g at birth.
  - Large for gestational age (LGA), small for gestational age (SGA), or intrauterine growth restriction (IUGR).
  - Infants of diabetic mothers.
  - < 37 or > 42 weeks' gestation at birth.
  - Suspected neonatal sepsis or maternal chorioamnionitis.
  - Apgar score < 7 at 5 minutes.
  - Newborns who required resuscitation.
  - Discordant twin (smaller).
  - Mother with limited prenatal care.
  - Cold stress or hypothermia.
  - Respiratory distress.

Watch out for:
- Symptoms of hypoglycemia including temperature instability, irritability or jitteriness, seizure activity, convulsions, exaggerated Moro reflex, high-pitched or weak cry, respiratory distress (e.g., grunting, flaring), irregular respiration, apnea, cynanosis, hypotonia, bradycardia, poor feeding, and lethargy (AAP Committee on Fetus and Newborn, 2011).
- The baby with hypoglycemia can be very lethargic and sleepy at the breast and may not exhibit obvious feeding cues.

What to do about it:
- Encourage mother to have as much skin-to-skin contact with baby as possible.
- Take a feeding history. Discover how the baby has been doing with breastfeeding—whether he or she has received supplementary feedings, and if so, what has been given.
- Observe a feeding using the feeding observation checklist (Appendix B).
- Assess adequacy of milk transfer (Appendix E).

Expected resolution:
- Hypoglycemia in the newborn is typically a short-term situation. The baby without underlying medical complications should be able to normalize blood sugar within a few hours of birth.
- Ongoing skin-to-skin contact and small amounts of colostrum obtained by licking and suckling at the breast typically assist the baby in normalizing the blood sugar within hours of birth.

What else to consider:
- Comprehensive pediatric evaluation if problems with hypoglycemia are not resolved by skin contact and feeding, and/or if signs of severe hypoglycemia are noted.

In Our Opinion

Skin-to-skin holding and feedings of colostrum are often underrated as first interventions for infants to prevent and treat hypoglycemia in an otherwise healthy baby. Fifteen minutes of skin-to-skin contact with the baby before a re-check of baby's glucose levels may increase the blood glucose levels to an acceptable number.

CONCERN: MY BABY HAS A BIRTH DEFECT

Descriptor: Presence of a Physiologic Anomaly in the Breastfed Baby

Presence of an anomaly does not mean that breastfeeding will be impossible.

Among the physiologic anomalies that may have an impact on breastfeeding are the following:

- *Cardiac (heart) defect.*
- Down syndrome.
- Craniofacial anomalies such as cleft lip, cleft palate, Pierre Robin sequence, and so on.
- Galactosemia.
- Phenylketonuria.

Unique Identifier: Baby Is Diagnosed with a Cardiac Problem

Ask yourself:

- What is the extent of the impact of the baby's condition on breastfeeding? Watch the baby at the breast to assess the baby's ability to seek the breast, latch, and transfer milk.

Watch out for:

- Babies with cardiac defects may fatigue easily at the breast, so they will need to be fed frequently.

- Observe for signs of cardiac problems, such as circumoral cyanosis during feeding.

What to do about it:
- Determine the feeding history—how the baby has been fed, how the baby is responding to feeding, and so on.
- Observe a feeding, using the feeding observation tool (Appendix B).
- If possible, collect pre- and postfeeding weight checks to quantify milk transfer (Appendix E).

Expected resolution:
- Cardiac defects have different degrees of impact on the ability to feed well in each baby affected. Many babies with cardiac problems can breast-feed well. However, they should be followed closely to ensure appropriate growth.

What else to consider:
- Many mothers of babies with cardiac problems will need to express milk after feeding to enhance milk removal (and thus milk supply).
- If baby does not transfer milk well during feedings, consider use of alternate massage (Appendix D) and/or at-breast supplementation with expressed breastmilk.

See also:
- Expression of breastmilk (Appendix M).
- Supplementary feeding devices (Appendix N).

In Our Opinion

Cardiac defects are among the most common birth defects, occurring in 1 in 100 births. Breast-feeding, or feeding expressed breastmilk in the event that feeding at the breast is not possible, can be a wonderful contribution to the health of the baby dealing with a heart problem.

CONCERN: MY BABY HAS A BIRTH DEFECT

Descriptor: Presence of a Physiologic Anomaly in the Breastfed Baby

Presence of an anomaly does not mean that breastfeeding will be impossible.

Among the physiologic anomalies that may have an impact on breastfeeding are the following:

- Cardiac (heart) defects.
- *Down syndrome.*
- Craniofacial anomalies such as cleft lip, cleft palate, Pierre Robin, and so on.
- Galactosemia.
- Phenylketonuria.

Unique Identifier: Baby Is Diagnosed with Down Syndrome

Ask yourself:
- What is the extent of the impact of the baby's condition on breastfeeding? Watch the baby at the breast to assess the baby's ability to seek the breast, latch, and transfer milk.

Watch out for:
- Babies with Down syndrome may fatigue easily at the breast, so they will need to be fed frequently.
- Babies with Down syndrome may have low muscle tone (as in **Figure 8-4**) that affects the baby's ability to create suction and draw milk from the breast, thus decreasing milk transfer, which can negatively affect mother's milk supply.
- Observe for signs of cardiac problems, such as circumoral cyanosis (blue tinge of the lips) during feeding. Babies with Down syndrome may also have heart or kidney problems.

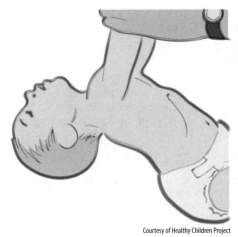

Courtesy of Healthy Children Project

Figure 8-4 The baby with low muscle tone (hypotonic) may not have the ability to pull the head up when lifted by the arms.

What to do about it:
- Determine the feeding history—how baby has been fed, how baby is responding to feeding, and so on.
- Observe a feeding, using the feeding observation tool (Appendix B).
- If possible, collect pre- and postfeeding weight checks to quantify milk transfer (Appendix E).

Expected resolution:
- Down syndrome has a different degree of impact on the ability to feed well in each baby it affects. Many babies with a diagnosis of Down syndrome can breastfeed well. However, they should be followed closely to ensure appropriate growth.

- Babies with Down syndrome become more proficient at breastfeeding with practice.

What else to consider:
- Many mothers of babies with Down syndrome will need to express milk after feeding to enhance milk removal (and thus milk supply).
- If baby does not transfer milk well during feedings, consider use of alternate massage (Appendix D) and/or at-breast supplementation with expressed breastmilk.

See also:
- Expression of breastmilk (Appendix M).
- Supplementary feeding devices (Appendix N).

In Our Opinion

It is well worth the clinician's time to support this family in breastfeeding. The many benefits of breastfeeding can be invaluable to this baby and this family, including reduced illness, increased IQ, enhanced bonding, and so on.

CONCERN: MY BABY HAS A BIRTH DEFECT

Descriptor: Presence of a Physiologic Anomaly in the Breastfed Baby

Presence of an anomaly does not mean that breastfeeding will be impossible.

Among the physiologic anomalies that may have an impact on breastfeeding are the following:

- Cardiac (heart) defects.
- Down syndrome.
- *Craniofacial anomalies such as cleft lip, cleft palate, Pierre Robin sequence, and so on.*
- Galactosemia.
- Phenylketonuria.

BABY FEEDING PROBLEMS

Unique Identifier: Baby Has Been Diagnosed with a Craniofacial Anomaly

Ask yourself:
- What is the extent of the impact of the baby's condition on breastfeeding? Watch the baby at the breast to assess the baby's ability to make a seal on the breast, keep the breast in the mouth, make and sustain a vacuum, and transfer milk.

Watch out for:
- Problems coordinating breathing and feeding.
- Signs of respiratory distress—for example, stridor (high-pitched noise when the baby inhales).
- Circumoral cyanosis (blue tinge of the lips) during feedings.

What to do about it:
- Determine the feeding history—how baby has been fed, how baby is responding to feeding, and so on.
- Observe a feeding, using the feeding observation tool (Appendix B).
- If possible, collect pre- and postfeeding weight checks to quantify milk transfer (Appendix E).
- With cleft lip, mother may be able to angle her breast so that the soft tissue fills the void in the lip. Alternatively, she may be able to close the lip area with her fingers.
- When dealing with a unilateral cleft palate, assist mother in angling her breast in the baby's mouth in such a way that the soft tissue of the breast fills the cleft area and the nipple extends into the intact side of the mouth.
- With Pierre Robin sequence, upright feeding posture may assist the baby in achieving deep latch.

Expected resolution:
- Babies with clefts and Pierre Robin sequence have varying degrees of success in feeding at the breast.

What else to consider:
- Many mothers of babies with these challenges will need to express milk after the feeding to maintain and increase their milk supply.
- If baby does not transfer milk well during feedings, consider use of alternate massage (Appendix D) and/or at-breast supplementation with expressed breastmilk.
- Special feeding devices that rely only on positive pressure to create milk flow have been used to feed babies who cannot transfer milk at the breast even when using an at-breast supplemental device.

See also:
- Milk expression (Appendix M).
- Supplementary feeding devices (Appendix N).
- Alternate massage (Appendix D).

In Our Opinion

In the event that a baby affected by one of these challenges is unable to feed at the breast, encourage the mother to continue to collect her milk to be fed to her baby. The baby will benefit from receiving mother's milk via any feeding method. In the event of a problem such as clefting, which will be surgically repaired, the baby may be able to breastfeed after the repair.

Concern: My Baby Has a Birth Defect

Descriptor: Presence of a Physiologic Anomaly in the Breastfed Baby

Presence of an anomaly does not mean that breastfeeding will be impossible.

Among the physiologic anomalies that may have an impact on breastfeeding are the following:

- Cardiac (heart) defects.
- Down syndrome.

Baby Feeding Problems

- Craniofacial anomalies such as cleft lip, cleft palate, Pierre Robin sequence, and so on.
- *Galactosemia (the inability of the body to use the simple sugar galactose, causing the accumulation of galactose 1-phosphate in the body, which results in damage to the liver, central nervous system, and other body systems with potentially permanent, even fatal, outcomes).*
- Phenylketonuria.

Unique Identifier: Baby Has Been Diagnosed with Galactosemia

Ask yourself:
- Has the baby been screened for galactosemia?
- Is the baby showing any signs of galactosemia prior to parents being notified about the results of a screening test?
- Is there a family history of galactosemia?

Watch out for:
- Jaundice, vomiting, poor feeding, poor weight gain, irritability, lethargy, convulsions, and opacity in the lenses of the eyes (all signs of galactosemia).

What to do about it:
- Determine which form of galactosemia has been diagnosed—classic or Duarte.
- Classic galactosemia is the sole pediatric contraindication to breastfeeding.
- Babies with Duarte galactosemia may be able to breastfeed, although some babies have both classic and Duarte forms of galactosemia.

Expected resolution:
- Breastfeeding is not recommended, except in individual cases of babies with Duarte galactosemia.
- Individuals with classic galactosemia must avoid all foods containing galactose (which occurs

naturally in all mammalian milks, including human milk as well as cow's milk-based formula, *including* those with reduced lactose). Consuming galactose will cause irreversible organ damage in the individual with galactosemia. A special formula is indicated.

What else to consider:
• Support the mother in decreasing her milk supply.

See also:
• Weaning.

In Our Opinion

These conditions are extremely rare. Classic galactosemia is thought to occur in 1 in 60,000 births. Duarte galactosemia is even rarer. When counseling the mother of a baby with classic galactosemia, allow space for her to express her feelings about the loss of the breastfeeding opportunity.

CONCERN: MY BABY HAS A BIRTH DEFECT

Descriptor: Presence of a Physiologic Anomaly in the Breastfed Baby

Presence of an anomaly does not mean that breastfeeding will be impossible.

Among the physiologic anomalies that may have an impact on breastfeeding are the following:

• Cardiac (heart) defects.
• Down syndrome.
• Craniofacial anomalies such as cleft lip, cleft palate, Pierre Robin sequence, and so on.
• Galactosemia.
• *Phenylketonuria (PKU)*.

Unique Identifier: Baby Has Been Diagnosed with Phenylketonuria

Ask yourself:
- Has the baby been screened for PKU?

Watch out for:
- Newborns do not have symptoms of PKU.
- Symptoms occurring in the first months may include eczema; jerking movements of arms and legs; rocking; tremors; seizures; hyperactivity; microcephaly; vomiting; and a musty odor in the child's breath, skin, or urine caused by too much phenylalanine in the body.

What to do about it:
- Discuss feeding plan with the pediatric care provider. Typically, babies with this disorder can be partially breastfed and are also fed a formula without phenylalanine. However, the volume of human milk consumed may need to be carefully monitored to ensure that levels of phenylalanine consumed are within safe limits. The baby will need some small amount of phenylalanine in the diet, which could come via breastfeeding.

Expected resolution:
- The outcome for babies with PKU is good, provided that levels of phenylalanine consumed can be kept low. If the baby's diet is not followed carefully, irreversible brain damage may result.

What else to consider:
- A team approach is best. The team should include at a minimum the lactation caregiver, the pediatric care provider, and the dietitian to monitor baby's progress.

See also:
• Weaning.

In Our Opinion

PKU is an uncommon disorder, occurring in 1 in every 15,000 births in the United States.

CONCERN: MY BABY HAS A BIRTH INJURY

Descriptor: Presence of a Birth Injury in the Breastfed Baby

• Presence of a birth injury does not mean that breastfeeding will be impossible.

Unique Identifier: Otherwise Intact Baby Who was Injured During the Birthing Process

Among the birth injuries that may have an impact on breastfeeding are the following:

• Cephalhematoma or caput succedaneum.
  ○ Cephalhematoma is a lump on the skull caused by bleeding beneath the bones of the skull. The lump arises within hours of birth.
  ○ Caput succedaneum is a swelling of the soft tissues of the baby's scalp that develops as the baby travels through the birth canal. This may occur when vacuum extraction is used to assist in birth.

Ask yourself:
• Does the baby cry or seem unable to feed when held in certain positions?
• Does holding or supporting the baby differently change the baby's ability to breastfeed?
• How is the mother supporting the baby's head? With this type of birth injury, there should be as little pressure on the head as possible.

Watch out for:
- People labeling the baby as hard to please or fussy.
- The mother feeling inadequate.
- Jaundice arising from resolving cephalohematoma (the baby's body reabsorbs the blood, increasing the amount of bilirubin in circulation).

What to do about it:
- Investigate what the family has been told about the condition.
- Determine the feeding history—how baby has been fed, how baby is responding to feeding, and so on.
- Observe a feeding, using the feeding observation tool (Appendix B).
- If baby is uncomfortable, try different feeding positions to attempt to take pressure off the injured area (Appendix C).

Expected resolution:
- Often, these conditions heal with time; however, physical therapy and other developmental interventions may be needed. Babies with brachial plexus injuries often have problems starting solid foods as well.

What else to consider:
- Comprehensive pediatric evaluation and occupational and/or physical therapy for the baby.
- Swallow study.

See also:
- Expression of breastmilk (Appendix M).

In Our Opinion

It is not surprising that babies with these conditions may not enjoy feeding. They probably have severe discomfort and pain. Pain relief may be prescribed for the baby who has noticeable discomfort.

CONCERN: MY BABY HAS A BIRTH INJURY

Descriptor: Presence of a Birth Injury in the Breastfed Baby

Presence of a birth injury does not mean that breastfeeding will be impossible.

Unique Identifier

Among the birth injuries that may have an impact on breastfeeding are the following:

- Fractured clavicle, brachial plexus injury, and so on.

Ask yourself:
- Does the baby cry or seem unable to feed when held in certain positions?
- Does holding or supporting the baby differently change the baby's ability to breastfeed?

Watch out for:
- People labeling the baby as hard to please.
- The mother feeling inadequate.
- Defining the situation as a "breastfeeding" problem and not seeking a medical diagnosis.
- Aspiration pneumonia.

What to do about it:
- Investigate what the family has been told about the condition.
- Determine the feeding history—how baby has been fed, how baby is responding to feeding, and so on.
- Observe a feeding, using the feeding observation tool (Appendix B).

- If baby is uncomfortable, try different positions to attempt to take pressure off the injured area (Appendix C). Babies with these conditions may feed best when lying flat on their back, which may require the use of pillows or other props to achieve comfort for the mother.
- A feeding study will determine if the baby is aspirating milk. Milk aspiration can lead to chemical pneumonia, which can be life threatening.

Expected resolution:
- Often, these conditions heal with time; however, physical therapy and other developmental interventions may be needed. Babies with brachial plexus injuries often have problems starting solid foods as well.

What else to consider:
- Comprehensive pediatric evaluation and occupational and/or physical therapy for the baby.
- Swallow study.

See also:
- Expression of breastmilk (Appendix M).

In Our Opinion

Babies with these injuries are often seen as problem breastfeeders and are changed to bottle feeding. In this event, use expressed breastmilk preferentially in the bottle. Feeding problems may reemerge when solid foods are tried and the baby chokes and gags.

CONCERN: MY BABY WAS BORN EARLY

Descriptor: Prematurity in the Breastfed Baby

Premature babies can have success with breastfeeding, but they may have a slow start.

Unique Identifier

Full-term pregnancy is considered to reflect babies born at and after 37 weeks of pregnancy. Babies born before that gestational age are considered to be premature. Babies born between the 34th and 37th weeks of pregnancy are referred to as late preterm infants.

Ask yourself:
- How is the mother's milk supply being supported?
- What is required regarding collection and storage of milk?
- What are the possibilities for skin-to-skin holding and practice breastfeedings?

Watch out for:
- Parents perceiving the baby as very fragile.
- The mother feeling inadequate.
- Difficulty regulating baby's heart rate, oxygenation, temperature, and breathing when breastfeeding.
- Concerns about adequacy of milk supply.

What to do about it:
- Investigate what the family knows about prematurity and the baby's ability to feed.
- Determine if baby has been stable enough to have skin-to-skin contact with parents.
- Determine the feeding history—how baby has been fed, how baby is responding to feeding, if baby is receiving human milk, if feeding is fortified, and so on.
- Explore the mother's milk expression plan and fine-tune as needed. For optimal results, milk expression should begin within 6 hours of birth and continue a minimum of 8 times in 24 hours to sustain adequate milk production when baby is not yet ready to feed at the breast.

BABY FEEDING PROBLEMS

- When baby is deemed ready for feeding at the breast, work with parents to establish reasonable expectations for the first feedings (for example, baby will lick or nuzzle at the breast rather than latch on and vigorous suckling). There is no specific age at which babies are "ready" for the breast. Coordination of the suck, swallow, breathe, and gag reflexes is important for safe oral feeding. The baby's ability to regulate cardiorespiratory stability should be the indicator that determines readiness for feeding at the breast (Nyqvist, Sjoden, & Ewald, 1999).
- Observe a feeding, using the feeding observation tool (Appendix B). Note that a special breastfeeding assessment tool is available for use with preterm infants (Phalen, 2011).
- Establish appropriate follow-up plans.

Expected resolution:
- Preterm babies grow in their feeding abilities with practice and the number of opportunities to try. The more time mother is able to spend with baby in skin-to-skin contact and practice breastfeedings, the faster baby will become adept at feeding.

What else to consider:
- Pediatric evaluation and referral to occupational and/or physical therapy for the baby.

See also:
- Expression of breastmilk (Appendix M).
- Collection and storage of breastmilk (Appendix P).
- Mother postures (Appendix C).
- Protocol for building the milk supply (Appendix J).

In Our Opinion

Preterm babies benefit greatly from receiving their mother's milk. Mother's milk is protective against necrotizing enterocolitis, a serious disorder common in preterm infants. Breast-feeding also allows the parents to observe the baby's innate abilities.

Along with all preterm babies, late preterm infants (LPTI) require special attention. While these babies are more likely to appear to have the capability of full-term infants, and to be cared for in the maternity unit rather than the NICU, they often seem to be sleepier, show fewer feeding cues and to have lower energy reserve. These factors may decrease the mother's milk production, and lead to low weight gain, or even weight loss for the LPTI. We encourage LCPs to observe these babies closely to determine if they are feeding adequately and effectively.

SECTION 9

Can She Breastfeed?

National and international health authorities concur that the vast majority of mothers and babies can breastfeed successfully (AAP, 2012; WHO, 2009). There are very few maternal and infant conditions that preclude breastfeeding (See Appendix Q for a current list.). Yet, the families of breastfed babies often worry about the appropriateness of human milk for their baby. In this section, we address some common questions families ask.

CONCERN: SMOKING AND BREASTFEEDING

Descriptor: Breastfeeding Woman Using Tobacco Cigarettes

Concerns have been raised about whether components of cigarette smoking can be found in breastmilk and what effect this might have on the baby.

Unique Identifier

Mother is concerned about choosing to breastfeed if she smokes.

Ask yourself:
- Is the mother aware of the need to protect the baby from all secondhand smoke?
- Did the mother smoke during pregnancy? If so, she should be encouraged to breastfeed and protect the baby from secondhand smoke. Research indicates that breastfeeding may mitigate the adverse effects on the child's cognitive

development of smoking during pregnancy
(Batstra, Neeleman, & Hadders-Algra, 2003).

- Is the mother willing to cut back on the number
  of cigarettes she smokes? Smokers may find some
  cigarettes more important than others (the first
  of the morning, after a meal, etc.); cutting those
  out can be easier.
- Is the mother motivated to stop smoking
  altogether? Perhaps there is a program that
  would work for her.
- Nicotine patches may be a choice for breastfeeding mothers who want to stop smoking. Nicotine
  gum does not lower the mother's blood levels of
  nicotine as well as the patch, and mothers may
  have fluctuations in blood levels not seen on the
  patch. Nicotine from a nicotine inhaler results in
  lower levels than inhaling cigarettes (Hale, 2014).

Watch out for:
- Fussiness. Babies of mothers who smoke may be
  fussier than other babies (Kelmanson, Erman, &
  Litvina, 2002).
- Mothers who smoke tend to nurse for fewer
  months than nonsmokers (K, & Platt, 2001).
- Mothers who smoke may make less milk than
  nonsmokers, possibly due to lower prolactin
  levels (Andersen et al., 1982).

What to do about it:
- It is accurate to say that tobacco components can
  be found in milk, but the greater exposure occurs
  if the mother smokes during pregnancy and/or if
  the baby is exposed to secondhand smoke.
- Cigarettes are very addictive. It may not be
  realistic to expect a mother to give up smoking
  to breastfeed.
- The benefits of receiving a smoking mother's
  milk outweigh any negatives.
- Emphasize the importance of protecting the baby
  from secondhand smoke.

- Help the mother think about her options for reducing or stopping smoking.
- Ensure frequent nursings and other good breastfeeding practices.
- Be familiar with local tobacco cessation resources, and ensure appropriate referrals.
- Ensure frequent weight checks for the baby.
- Help the mother with baby's fussiness if that becomes an issue.

Expected resolution:
- Even if a mother continues to smoke, she should be encouraged to breastfeed, if that is what she wants to do.
- The baby must be protected from secondhand smoke no matter whether feeding by breast or formula.

In Our Opinion

More effort should be expended helping parents understand the importance of protecting babies from secondhand smoke and the disadvantages of formula feeding than on the possible cigarette toxins conveyed to the baby via breastmilk.

CONCERN: MOTHER TAKING AN OVER-THE-COUNTER OR PRESCRIPTION MEDICATION

Descriptor: Safety of Medications During Breastfeeding

Most medications likely to be prescribed to the nursing mother have little effect on milk supply or on infant well-being, although there are some categories of drugs such as antimetabolites and street drugs (recreational/illegal substances) that are always contraindicated. Radioactive compounds usually require a temporary cessation of breastfeeding that varies according to the compound.

Medications (including prescription and over-the-counter preparations as well as vitamins, nutritional supplements, and herbal remedies) should be checked with a reliable source:

- The United States National Library of Medicine maintains LactMed, a peer-reviewed and fully referenced database of drugs to which breastfeeding mothers may be exposed. Among the data included are maternal and infant levels of drugs, possible effects on breastfed infants and on lactation, and alternate drugs to consider (Appendix Y). A smartphone application is available for this service.
- The reference book *Medications and Mother's Milk*, written by Thomas Hale, PhD, is a comprehensive reference on the impact of currently used medications on breastfeeding mothers and infants. Updated biannually, this resource has an easy-to-use rating system (Hale, 2014). A smartphone application is available for this text as well (fee applies).
- The Infant Risk Center is an Internet and telephone resource based on Dr. Hale's work (Appendix Y).
- From time to time, the AAP publishes a list of prescription and nonprescription drugs, indicating their compatibility with breastfeeding (Sachs & Committee on Drugs, 2013).

Unique Identifier

The name of the medication or substance, dosage, route of administration, age of baby.

Ask yourself:
- If the medication is one that is of concern for breastfeeding mothers, can a different, more appropriate medication be substituted?

- If the medication is of the "long-acting" type, can a "short-acting" one be substituted?
- If the mother has to take a contraindicated medication, what plan can be made to keep up her milk supply or help her wean? What is the plan for feeding the baby?

Watch out for:
- Recommendations made to mothers that are not evidence-based, because uninformed prescribers may have the mistaken idea that mothers cannot breastfeed if they take any medication.
- Mothers who do not take prescribed medication because they think that it may be contraindicated.
- Assuming drugs that are considered safe during pregnancy are also safe during lactation. This is not always the case.
- Babies who have otherwise unexplained behaviors.

What to do about it:
- Ensure appropriate resources for mothers and prescribers so that evidence-based decisions can be made.

Expected resolution:
- With few exceptions, breastfeeding and medications are compatible.

What else to consider:
- Changes in milk supply. For example, pseudoephedrine has been shown to reduce milk supply (Aljazaf et al., 2003).
- Baby behavior (some drugs [such as tricyclics] accumulate over time and may make baby drowsy and sleepy).
- Other effects on the baby (for example, fluoxetine has been associated with slower growth in the baby).

In Our Opinion

While there are occasions when a mother cannot breastfeed because of a contraindicated medication, they are quite rare. Unfortunately, many women end up weaning unnecessarily due to inadequate knowledge about medication safety. The potential side effects of receiving breastmilk substitutes are rarely considered in this equation, as Amir (2007) has identified.

Be prepared to provide clinicians with resources for current, evidence-based, information regarding medications and breastfeeding.

CONCERN: MOTHER IS ILL

Descriptor: Safety of Breastfeeding During Maternal Illness

The mother could have an illness that is acute or chronic, infective or noninfective. Different countries have their own recommendations, especially for HIV-positive mothers or for women who are at high risk for HIV (Appendix Q).

Unique Identifier

Maternal health conditions may impact breastfeeding, but few are absolute contraindications to breastfeeding. (See also Appendix Q for a more concise chart from the Centers for Disease Control and Prevention [CDC])

- In the United States, HIV-positive and HTLV-I–or HTLV-II–positive women should be advised not to breastfeed.
- Women with acute infectious diseases such as respiratory, reproductive, or gastrointestinal infections may breastfeed.
- Women with active tuberculosis may breastfeed after 2 or more weeks of treatment. Tuberculosis

is communicated via droplets, not mother's milk, so the mother will be separated from her baby but may collect her milk to be fed to the baby by someone else.

- Women with hepatitis A may breastfeed as soon as they have received gamma globulin.
- Women with hepatitis B may breastfeed. The infant should receive hepatitis B immune globulin (HBIG) and the first dose of hepatitis B vaccine within 12 hours of birth. There is no reason to delay breastfeeding (CDC, 2009b).
- Women with hepatitis C may breastfeed. However, the CDC (2009b) advises that breastfeeding women with cracked, bleeding nipples abstain from nursing on the bleeding nipple until healing occurs.
- Women with venereal warts may breastfeed.
- For the herpes viruses:
  - For cytomegalovirus (CMV), breastfeeding the full-term infant is allowed. For premature babies, the AAP's Section on Breastfeeding (2012) states that freezing milk reduces but does not eliminate CMV, and that fresh mothers' own milk is the preferred food for all pre-term infants.
  - For herpes simplex, breastfeeding is allowed, except if the lesion is on the breast, areola, or nipple.
  - For varicella-zoster, chicken pox, the mother may breastfeed when she is noninfectious.
  - For Epstein-Barr, breastfeeding is allowed.
- Mothers with toxoplasmosis and mastitis may breastfeed.
- Mothers with Lyme disease may breastfeed as soon as treatment is initiated.
- Mothers with untreated brucellosis should not breastfeed or provide milk for their babies (AAP Section on Breastfeeding, 2012).

- Since flu viruses are changing rapidly, caregivers for mothers acutely infected with influenza should verify the safety of mother-baby contact and breastfeeding with their state health department and/or the CDC.

Ask yourself:
- Are the drugs prescribed for the condition contraindicated for breastfeeding mothers?
- What other support does the mother need to cope with her condition?

Watch out for:
- Ideas that mothers who are ill should be separated from their baby and that every ill mother will convey the illness through her breastmilk and/or breastfeeding. This is not always the case.

What to do about it:
- Consult with state health departments, the CDC, or other national infectious disease authorities when there are questions about breastfeeding and illness or disease (Appendix Y).
- Each case must be assessed individually. Contraindications to breastfeeding are rare.
- Be prepared to identify sources of evidence-based, up-to-date information about safety of breastfeeding to clinicians working with breastfeeding families.

What else to consider:
- Contraindications to breastfeeding (Appendix Q).

In Our Opinion

Contact information for your state or provincial health departments, the CDC, and other health authorities are important resources to have at your fingertips. When questions arise about possible contraindications, mothers need immediate, reliable answers.

CONCERN: BREASTFEEDING MOTHER IS PREGNANT

Descriptor: Breastfeeding During Pregnancy

Unique Identifier

Mother becomes pregnant while breastfeeding.

Ask yourself:
- Does the mother have a history of premature delivery, miscarriage, or threatened premature delivery? If so, the oxytocin-mediated uterine contractions associated with breastfeeding are a concern. There is no compelling research that would indicate that low-risk mothers should wean. In fact, a recent Japanese study found no increased risk of miscarriage or preterm labor in a group of women continuing to nurse through pregnancy compared with those who weaned prior to conception (Ishii, 2009).
- Does the mother have sore nipples? Some mothers who have a desire to continue breastfeeding throughout the pregnancy may find that nipple soreness is so uncomfortable that they cannot continue.
- Is the baby less than 1 year old? Will the baby be under 1 year when the mother is 4 to 5 months pregnant? Mothers often find that the volume of milk decreases as mature milk becomes colostral in mid-pregnancy. Nutrition assessment of the baby's intake will be needed to determine if the baby will need formula supplementation.

Watch out for:
- Appropriate nutrition for the mother and the nursling.
- Some babies have very loose stools when the milk becomes colostral (this is not because the milk is "bad," but because colostrum is a powerful laxative).

- Many worry that the new baby will get less colostrum because the older baby takes it all during the pregnancy. This has not been found to be a problem, as the hormones of pregnancy trigger continued synthesis of colostrum until complete delivery of the placenta occurs.

What to do about it:
- Support the mother in her choice to continue breastfeeding or to wean.
- Ensure adequate nutrition for mother, the nursling, and the new baby.

Expected resolution:
- Some mothers decide to wean when they learn that they are pregnant.
- Others continue nursing throughout the pregnancy.
- Others nurse both babies together. Nursing two babies not from the same pregnancy is called tandem nursing.
  - The new baby should be fed first and often.
  - Mother should work to find time for non-breastfeeding interactions with the older baby.

What else to consider:
- Some mothers find that they want to nurse during pregnancy and go on to tandem breastfeed, but the older baby loses interest when the volume decreases as milk changes mid-pregnancy.
- Some mothers wonder if they should offer a weaned older baby an opportunity to breastfeed after the new baby is born. We advise mothers to think very carefully about the ramifications of this offer before making it. Many formerly breastfed children may have forgotten how to release milk from the breast, but the mother should be prepared for the possibility that her weaned child does recall how to trigger milk flow and wants to

return to breastfeeding. Would that be acceptable to the mother?

In Our Opinion

The improved nutrition of mothers today has made breastfeeding during pregnancy and tandem nursing viable options for many mothers.

CONCERN: WEANING

Descriptor: Beginning Other Foods or Stopping Breastfeeding

Unique Identifier

The end of breastfeeding this baby. Weaning can be characterized as one of three types:

- Mother-led weaning, where the mother makes the decision to end breastfeeding (most of the following discussion refers to this type of weaning).
- Baby-led weaning, where the mother goes to a breastfeeding "on-request-only" system and uses the philosophy, "Never offer but never refuse." This is only for babies more than 1 year old. The idea is that the baby gets so involved in a busy life that breastfeeding takes a more minor role.
- Society-led weaning, where everyone in the society weans at the same time (usually after the second year). Weaning is a time for ritual and celebration.

Ask yourself:
- What do I mean when I use the word *wean*? What does this mother mean?
  ○ For some people, the word *wean* means beginning to stop breastfeeding. For others, wean means that breastfeeding has stopped

altogether. Yet others mean continuing to breastfeed while adding complementary foods. It is important to know that you and the mother are using the word in the same way.

○ For example, the mother may say, "I'm ready to wean my baby." She could mean, "I want to start feeding my baby other foods besides my milk." Or she could mean, "I want today to be the last time I breastfeed." Or she could mean, "I would like my baby to drop the nighttime nursing."

• If the mother wants to stop breastfeeding altogether, how fast does she want this to happen? In 1 day? In 3 months? By the time the baby is 1 or 2 years old? Rapid weaning can have negative consequences for the mother (such as breast discomfort, mastitis, and abscess development) and the baby (for example, longing for nursing or no longer being potty trained). The faster the weaning, the more watchful she will need to be.

Watch out for:

• Choice of breastmilk substitutes. What is appropriate to replace mother's milk? For babies under 1 year, formula is the appropriate substitute. How does the baby react to the substitute? Are there any physical reactions?

• Choice of breastfeeding substitute. The substitute for the closeness of breastfeeding has to be equally good in the eyes of the child. Asking a 9-month-old baby to wean from a breastfeeding by crying it out alone in a crib is obviously not an equal substitute, but having a fun bath time with Daddy, a sippy cup of water, or a healthy snack might be.

• Speed of weaning. It is possible to stop breastfeeding quickly, but the breasts do not stop making milk quickly. Depending on her stage of lactation and milk volume, the mother may need to continue to remove milk and gradually decrease her milk supply to prevent engorgement, mastitis, and abscess.

- Emotional responses. With baby-led weaning, sometimes the baby is less interested in continuing the nursing relationship than the mother; the mother may feel wistful about the loss of their special time together. With mother-led weaning, the baby may feel rejected or ignored and shut down, or become demanding.

What to do about it:
- Sometimes mothers who did not need any help to breastfeed are surprised at how much help and support they need during weaning.
- Sometimes mothers stop breastfeeding and the baby cannot tolerate the substitute. See Appendix J for information about relactation.

Expected resolution:
- The mother will remember her breastfeeding time and the weaning time with joy, irrespective of the duration.

What else to consider:
- Do not confuse weaning with a nursing strike, which is a sudden refusal of the baby to nurse even though the mother has plenty of milk.
  - Strikes are not the same as weaning, but some strikes are never resolved and signal an end to breastfeeding. Babies under year of age rarely wean intentionally.
  - There are many reasons for a nursing strike; for example:
    - Baby cannot nurse because of a stuffy nose.
    - Baby is teething.
    - Baby has an ear infection.
    - Baby prefers bottle.
    - Baby has bitten mother and mother responded by yelling, scaring the baby.
    - Family stress.
    - Separation.

○ The problem has to be dealt with before the baby will return to nursing.
○ Assist the mother with temporary milk expression and alternative feeding method (e.g. cup, spoon, etc.) to deliver milk to the baby.
- To end the strike:
  ○ Offer lots of skin-to-skin contact.
  ○ Never force a baby to the breast.
  ○ If possible, avoid bottles.
  ○ Try offering the breast when the baby is sleepy.
  ○ Try bringing the baby to a nursing mother's meeting; babies may respond to the peer pressure of seeing other nursing babies.
- Sometimes a mother begins weaning and then changes her mind. Her milk supply can be built up again if need be.
- Some people think that the only reason a mother is nursing a baby for more than 6 months is because she does not know how to wean and may subject her to unkind remarks.

In Our Opinion

In the United States, public nursing of babies older than 6 months is rare, so mothers may think they are supposed to wean because they only see young babies nursing in public. As breastfeeding becomes more of the cultural norm and is seen more in public, it is our hope that the duration of breastfeeding will increase.

CONCERN: BIRTH CONTROL
Descriptor: Avoiding Pregnancy While Breastfeeding
Unique Identifier

Birth control or family planning methods compatible with breastfeeding.

Ask yourself:
- What are the mother's plans for future pregnancies?
- How do her religious beliefs, health concerns, or lifestyle preferences affect her choices for family planning?
- What choices are more or less appropriate for breastfeeding mothers?

Watch out for:
- Misunderstanding the relationship between breastfeeding and fertility. Some people believe that you can't get pregnant when breastfeeding— not true!
- Hormonal methods of birth control containing estrogen. These are not recommended in early lactation (Centers for Disease Control and Prevention, 2011a).
- Starting progestin-only types of birth control too early. For example, the package insert for Depo-Provera suggests starting in the 6th week postpartum in breastfeeding women.

What to do about it:
- Progestin-only forms of birth control are options for nursing mothers after the early weeks. These include birth control pills, injections, and implants.
- All barrier methods, including cervical caps, condoms, diaphragms, foam, and so on, are acceptable for nursing mothers. (Note that most nursing mothers have vaginal dryness and are more comfortable having intercourse when additional lubrication is used.)
- Carefully explore the options with each mother, including the lactational amenorrhea method (LAM) (See **Figure 9-1.**). Research studies indicate that the cumulative pregnancy rate using LAM is similar to other types of birth control (Kennedy, 2002).

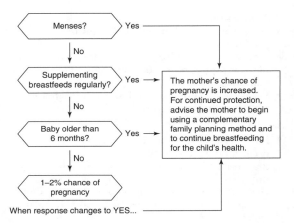

Figure 9-1 Lactational Amenorrhea Method (LAM).
Modified from Labbok, M., Cooney, K., & Coly, S. (1994).
Guidelines: Breastfeeding, family planning, and the Lactational Amenorrhea Method—LAM. Washington, DC: Institute for Reproductive Health.

Expected resolution:
- The mother will find a method of birth control or child spacing that meets her needs and is compatible with breastfeeding.

What else to consider:
- Learn about the availability of books and classes for parents on other methods of child spacing, such as the symptothermal method (or Natural Family Planning), a combination of calendar rhythm, basal body temperature, and other techniques.

In Our Opinion

Birth control options are not thoroughly discussed with mothers in relation to breastfeeding plans, so mothers may think that breastfeeding is not compatible with birth control—not true!

CONCERN: BREASTFEEDING MULTIPLE BABIES—TWINS, TRIPLETS, AND MORE

Descriptor: Breastfeeding Multiples

Women who give birth to multiple babies may be concerned about whether breastfeeding is possible. Women can make enough milk for many babies, but the situation is often complicated by prematurity and concerns about milk supply.

Unique Identifier

Mother wants to breastfeed twins, triplets, or other multiples.

Ask yourself:
- Were the babies born prematurely?
- Was the mother on bed rest? Mothers who have been on bed rest may have muscle atrophy and fatigue easily. This does not influence milk supply, but it does influence the mother's ability to cope with the stress of multiple, often premature, babies.
- Are the babies able to transfer milk?
- What resources, physical and emotional, are available to the family?

Watch out for:
- Lethargy.
- Decrease in urine and stools.
- Change in breastfeeding behavior.
- Problems with feeding.

What to do about it:
- Nursing babies simultaneously is helpful for building a milk supply, but may be difficult to manage at first. Offer help with positioning. A variety of positions, shown in **Figure 9-2**, work well with multiples.

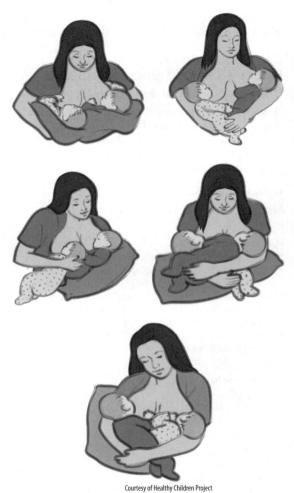

Courtesy of Healthy Children Project

Figure 9-2 There are several positions that work well for simultaneous feeding.

- At first, switch the babies from one breast to the other. As the babies get older, they may prefer nursing on one breast or the other.
- Many mothers have found it helpful at first to write down "who" nursed "when" to be sure that each baby gets enough.
- Undertake a feeding assessment (Appendix B).

Expected resolution:
- There is no way to know ahead of time how much milk a mother will be able to make. Frequent weight checks of the babies are needed to assess growth in the early weeks.

What else to consider:
- Encourage the mother to keep an open mind about the babies' feeding plan. Some mothers who planned to pump and feed bottles some of the time find that feeding only at the breast is easier.

In Our Opinion

Simultaneous nursing is very helpful to ensuring an adequate milk supply. It is important to have weekly or more frequent weight checks of the babies to ensure that all of the babies are thriving, especially with higher order multiples (three or more babies). There is no reason to suspect that a mother cannot make enough milk for multiples, given adequate stimulation, milk removal, and support.

APPENDIX A

The Healthy Children Eight-Level Breastfeeding Counseling Process

DESCRIPTION OF THE PROCESS

The eight-level breastfeeding counseling process, depicted in **Figure A-1**:

- Combines the use of empirical knowledge with critical thinking skills.
- Helps refine choice of solutions from a sea of possibilities.
- Develops a broader vision of compassionate service to mothers and babies.

Each level must be addressed; skipping or only partially addressing a level can lead to wrong, incomplete, or inadequate resolution of breast-feeding problems.

Level 1: Take a complete history
Level 2: Assess the mother, the baby, and the feeding
Level 3: Develop a symptom list
Level 4: Formulate a problem list
Level 5: Reconcile the history, assessment, symptoms, and problems
Level 6: Generate and prioritize solutions and plans for interventions
Level 7: Reconcile prioritized solutions and planned interventions with problems
Level 8: Evaluate solutions and interventions

APPLYING THE PROCESS

The purpose of applying the counseling process is to ensure that in every case empirical knowledge is combined with critical thinking skills.

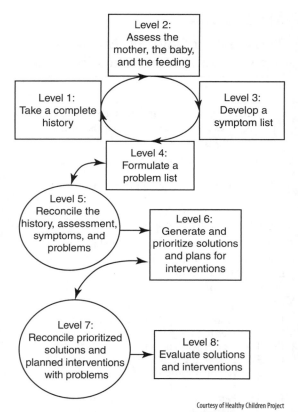

Courtesy of Healthy Children Project

Figure A-1 The eight-level lactation consulting process.

The first four levels are interactive with each other. If you look at the diagram of the process in Figure A-1, you can see that we picture these levels as being connected by a series of arrows that go around in a circular motion. That's because the nature of the process is interactive. These four levels are rarely completed in order, one after another. Instead, the lactation care provider must multitask, moving fluidly among each of the first four levels. The activity of assessment of the feeding, for example, should not be forced. If the observer instructs the mother to begin to feed, the prefeeding interaction of the mother and baby may be missed. If the history is completed first, the baby could be crying and frantic by the time the nursing starts.

The counselor must be present in the moment, noting behavior, asking questions, and critically thinking: "What else do I need to know?", "What is missing from the history, symptoms, and assessment that keeps me from identifying a problem that unites the findings?"

There are two levels shown as circles in Figure A-1: Level 5 and Level 7. These are the levels at which we stop and consider what we know and how we know what we know. This is where we ask ourselves, "Does what I'm thinking make sense?" These two levels are essential to ensure the highest quality of care for the mothers and babies we serve. At Level 5, we stop and reconcile the history, assessment, symptoms, and problems we have formulated. To generate and prioritize solutions and plans for interventions (Level 6), we must be sure that the problems we have formulated reconcile with the history, assessment, and symptoms. Ask yourself if other assessments should be made that are outside your scope of practice and require a referral to another provider for more information. Diagnostic tests? If you had more time, would your assessment be different?

Like Level 5, Level 7 is one where we stop and reconcile our thinking. Do the solutions we have planned integrate appropriately with the problem(s) we have formulated? We ask ourselves if our solutions are evidence-based. We ask if the solutions have been shown to be effective for each of the problems we have formulated. Do any of the solutions contradict each other? Will any solution or intervention cause harm? Use up-to-date breastfeeding texts and research articles to guide your selection of targeted solutions and interventions. Be sure to read any information thoroughly. Ask yourself if there are any exceptions to the intervention or solution. Look up words in the index in the back of this book to see if there is additional information in another section of the book that might make a difference for this mother and baby.

Ask yourself also whether the plans and solutions you have prioritized are within your scope of practice to recommend. Is a referral to another practitioner needed? Have you compromised the outcome for the mother and baby by not working with other members of the healthcare team? An example of this is the recommendation of a home remedy when a prescription may result in a better outcome.

Levels 5 and 7 are also the two levels at which we are mandated to stop and check with the mother about what we are thinking. We tell the mother what we think the problems are and why they make sense to us based on the history, assessment, and symptoms. Do they make sense to her? We have had mothers tell us that we misunderstood symptoms or history, that they don't feel comfortable about our problem formulation, or that they would like us to assess something else. Again at Level 7, we discuss the way we are thinking with the mother. This is the level where we may discover that she does not want to nurse more often, pump, or use an at-breast feeding system. She may tell us that she's confused, it seems like too much work, she doesn't feel confident, or she doesn't have transportation. It is also the level at which she can agree with our plan. Level 7, like Level 5, if skipped or rushed, can have disastrous results not only because of the "buy-in" from the mother, but because of the critical thinking that is part of each of these two levels.

Examples of the eight-level counseling process as applied to breastfeeding situations have been previously published (Cadwell & Turner-Maffei, 2004).

APPENDIX B

Feeding Observation Checklist

Before the feed:

☐ If possible, weigh baby prior to feeding on a digital scale, sensitive to 2 grams. Baby need not be naked, but should be weighed after the feeding in the same clothes, without diaper changing.

☐ Does skin-to-skin contact precede the feeding?

☐ What cues does mother respond to in deciding when to feed?

☐ Is the baby too hungry to feed well (for example, frantic, crying)?

☐ Is the baby not hungry at all (for example, deeply sleeping, shut down)?

☐ How does mother prepare for the feed?

☐ How much time lapses from observed cues until baby is brought to the breast?

☐ Position yourself so that you can best view the feeding from the mother's perspective. For example, standing behind the mother or beside the mother.

As the baby latches:

☐ What does the nipple look like before it enters the baby's mouth? Note shape and coloration.

☐ What position does the mother choose?

☐ Is baby's body turned toward mother?

☐ Is baby's body aligned (ears over shoulders, shoulders over hips, legs and arms flexed to midline)?

☐ Where are mother's hands?

☐ Does she have her hand on the back of the baby's head or the sides of the baby's face?

☐ Is she using her hand to alter the natural shape of the breast and/or the tilt of the nipple?

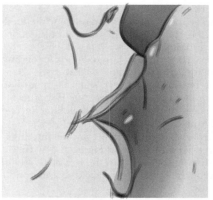

Courtesy of Healthy Children Project

Figure B-1 Baby's mouth is latched to the breast at a 90-degree angle.

☐ What is baby's position relative to the mother's nipple?
☐ When does baby open mouth?
☐ What is the angle of mouth opening? For example, the baby in **Figure B-1** has a mouth opening angle of approximately 90 degrees, too small for effective, comfortable feeding.
☐ Does mother respond to wide-open mouth by drawing baby in close?
☐ Is baby able to extend the head backward? Or is the head being held toward the baby's chest?
☐ Does baby reach breast with lower lip and tongue first, followed by the upper lip sealing to the breast?
☐ Does baby's mouth appear off-center in relation to the position of the nipple?
☐ Is baby's chin dug into the breast?
☐ Is baby's nose near the breast?
☐ Are the baby's arms up around (hugging) the breast?

During the feed:

☐ Observe mother's body language while feeding. Look for tension in arms, shoulders, hands, feet, and face.

☐ Observe baby's body language while feeding. Look for signs of tension or distress.

☐ Is the motion of the baby's jaw an up-and-down piston motion as in **Figure B-2**? If so, this is correlated with nonnutritive sucking and poor milk transfer.

☐ Is the motion of the baby's jaw moving in a rocker-like fashion as in **Figure B-3**, with the jaw driving forward into the breast? If so, this is correlated with nutritive sucking and good milk transfer.

☐ How does baby handle the milk flow?

☐ Does baby sputter or choke during the feeding?

☐ Does baby release the breast in order to take a breath?

☐ Does baby stay at the breast or come off and on during the feed?

☐ Does baby seem to have difficulty breathing at the breast?

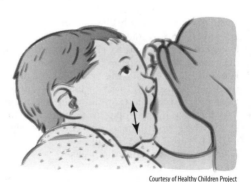

Courtesy of Healthy Children Project

Figure B-2 Piston motion of the jaw is associated with nonnutritive sucking.

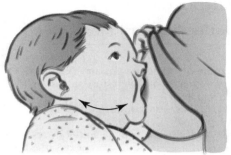

Courtesy of Healthy Children Project

Figure B-3 Rocker motion of the jaw is ideal and associated with nutritive sucking.

☐ Does the skin around the baby's mouth and nose appear normal during the feeding? (Blue coloration is a sign of a medical problem—ensure immediate comprehensive pediatric exam.)

☐ Count rhythm of sucks to swallows. Expect bursts of one suck to one swallow, or two sucks to one swallow.

After the feed:

☐ What triggers the end of the feed (the clock, the mother's determination that the feed is over, or the baby's self-removal)?

☐ What does the mother's nipple look like just as it exits the baby's mouth? Any change in shape (other than increased length and width)?

☐ Any change in coloration of the nipple?

APPENDIX C

Breastfeeding Positions

The cradle or Madonna posture (Figure C-1):
- The mother sits in any posture that is comfortable.
- The baby lies on his or her side, facing the mother.
- The side of the baby's head and body rest on the mother's forearm, of the arm next to the breast being used.

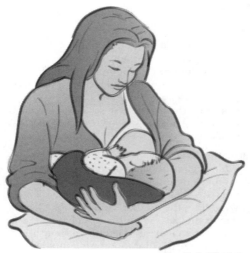

Courtesy of Healthy Children Project

Figure C-1 In the cradle posture, the mother supports the baby with the same arm as the breast the baby is nursing from.

The cross-cradle posture (Figure C-2):

This position is considered especially useful for the mother of a newborn or preterm infant:

- The mother sits in any posture that is comfortable.
- The infant lies on his or her side, facing the mother.
- The side of the infant's body rests on the mother's forearm, of the arm on the opposite side of the breast being used.
- The hand supports the baby's neck and shoulders in such a way that the baby can tilt his or her head.

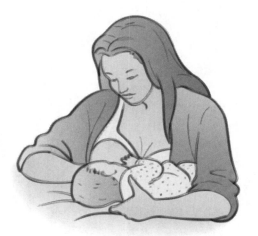

Courtesy of Healthy Children Project

Figure C-2 Using the cross-cradle posture, the mother holds the baby with the arm opposite the breast. Note that the mother's hand is not putting pressure against the back of the baby's head.

The football or clutch posture (Figure C-3):
- The mother sits in any posture that is comfortable.
- The infant lies on his or her back, curled between the side of the mother's chest and her arm.
- The infant's upper body is supported by the mother's forearm.
- The mother's hand supports the infant's neck and shoulders, without pressing on the back of the head.
- The infant's hips are flexed along the chair's back or any other surface the mother is leaning against.

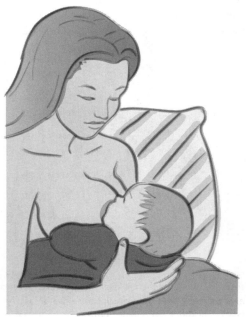

Courtesy of Healthy Children Project

Figure C-3 In the football posture, the baby's legs extend under the mother's arm.

The semi-reclining (or "laid-back") posture (Figure C-4):
- The mother sits in a comfortable, semi-reclining posture.
- The mother leans back and the baby lies against her body, usually prone.

The side-lying posture (Figure C-5):
- The mother lies on her side.
- The infant is placed on his or her side, lying chest to chest with mother.
- The mother's arm closest to the mattress or a rolled blanket supports the infant's back.

The Australian posture (Figure C-6):
- The mother is "down under," lying on her back.
- The baby is supported on her chest.
- This position is useful when the mother has a large milk supply or a powerful let-down because the baby has more ability to maneuver his or her head to better manage rapid milk flow.

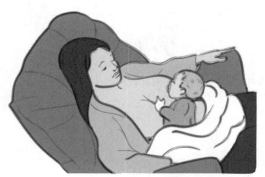

Courtesy of Healthy Children Project

Figure C-4 In the semi-reclining posture, the baby is supported on the mother's body. Note that the baby's head and body are free to move.

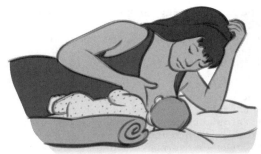

Courtesy of Healthy Children Project

Figure C-5 Mothers can nurse lying down.

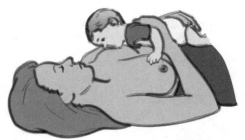

Courtesy of Healthy Children Project

Figure C-6 When using the Australian posture, the mother is "down under."

Alternate Massage/Breast Compression

Alternate massage or breast compression is a technique to increase the flow of milk. The mother uses her hand to compress or massage her breast when the baby is not sucking (hence the term alternate massage, shown in **Figure D-1**).

This technique is especially useful with a baby who sucks a few times and then has a long pause.

The mother can use massage/compression to increase the flow of milk, which will stimulate the baby to nurse actively again. This works especially well with premies, babies with Down

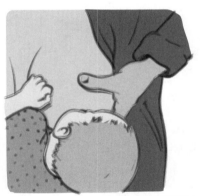

Courtesy of Healthy Children Project

Figure D-1 Alternate massage or breast compression is a way to increase the flow of milk to the baby. The mother compresses the breast when the baby pauses.

195

syndrome, and other babies who are weak or impaired.

Mothers who are nursing a baby with a cleft palate use a more active alternate massage because the baby usually cannot maintain a vacuum. Her hand action is similar to manual expression (Appendix M). The mother develops a synchronicity with the baby's sucking, increasing the flow of milk so that the baby can manage a greater flow.

APPENDIX E

Protocol for Estimating Breastmilk Transfer

- Obtain a prefeeding weight on an accurate digital scale sensitive to 2 grams.
  - To check the accuracy of a scale, use a standard weight. These are available from scale manufacturers.
  - To check whether a digital scale can accurately measure 2 grams, put a book on the scale. Note the weight. Add a U.S. quarter (25-cent coin). If the scale registers the additional weight of the quarter, it measures accurately.
- Observe a feeding using the feeding observation checklist (Appendix B).
- Observe baby's approach to the breast. Does baby exhibit interest in feeding? Does baby seem to be conserving energy or actively feeding? When baby is attached to the breast, observe for sucking and swallowing.
- If baby stops suckling and appears to go to sleep, ask the mother to use alternate massage to change the rate of flow of the milk. Observe for sucking and swallowing. Does baby get more wakeful and suckle more actively, or does baby break suction?
- Conduct a postfeeding weight check. Calculate milk transfer. (The increase in grams of weight equates to milk volume transferred by the baby at that feeding.) Calculate the baby's approximate daily needs (Appendix F) and divide that figure by the amount of reported feeds in 24 hours.

- Note: Any one feeding does not necessarily indicate a typical milk intake. For this reason, it is helpful to observe several feedings over a period of time to get a better estimate of average transfer. Also, try different positions (e.g., cross-cradle, semi-reclining, football) to determine if there is better transfer in one or the other.

APPENDIX F

Protocol to Calculate Baby's Approximate Daily Needs

Several methods have been used to calculate a baby's approximate daily needs, with the understanding that there may be a variation from baby to baby, nursing to nursing, and day to day.

Note: Any one feeding does not necessarily indicate a typical milk intake. For this reason, it is helpful to observe several feedings over a period of time to get a better estimate of average transfer. Also, try different positions (e.g., cross-cradle, semi-reclining, football) to determine if there is better transfer in one or the other.

The method we use at the Center for Breastfeeding is to take the baby's weight in pounds and multiply by 2.5 for standard gain and 2.7 to 3.0 if the baby needs to catch up on weight. These standard multipliers are based on the AAP's (2011) calculations for intake of formula-fed babies and may not correctly predict the breastfed baby's needs. They are just a rough calculation of potential need and are likely to be most accurate for the newborn baby.

Note: The determination of which multiplier (2.5, 2.7, or 3.0) is made by the pediatric care provider.

So, for an 8-pound baby who is gaining well:

$$8 \times 2.5 = 20 \text{ ounces per day}$$

If the 8-pound baby is not gaining well:

$$8 \times 2.7 = 21.6 \text{ ounces per day}$$

or

$$8 \times 3 = 24 \text{ ounces per day}$$

Appendix G provides a table of milk requirements, catch-up requirements at 2.7, and catch-up requirements at 3 times the baby's weight.

Example

Baby weighs 6 pounds.

$$6 \times 2.5 = 15 \text{ ounces}$$
(expected daily intake)

Mother reports 10 breastfeedings
per day:

15 ounces ÷ 10 feedings a day = approximately
1.5 ounces per feeding

Before and after weights show an intake of 0.5 ounce for one breastfeeding. Conclusion: During this feed, the baby transferred much less milk than we would expect. Further evaluation of milk supply and feeding effectiveness is needed (Appendices J, L).

APPENDIX G-1

Table of Daily Breastmilk Volume Requirement Estimates (in Ounces)

BABY WEIGHT (LB-OZ)	REQUIRED MILK (2.5)	CATCH-UP MILK 1 (2.7)	CATCH-UP MILK 2 (3.0)
5-0	12.5	13.5	15.0
5-1	12.69	13.69	15.19
5-2	12.81	13.81	15.38
5-3	13.0	14.0	15.56
5-4	13.13	14.19	15.75
5-5	13.31	14.38	15.94
5-6	13.44	14.5	16.13
5-7	13.63	14.69	16.31
5-8	13.75	14.88	16.5
5-9	13.94	15.0	16.69
5-10	14.06	15.19	16.88
5-11	14.25	15.38	17.06
5-12	14.38	15.5	17.25
5-13	14.56	15.69	17.44
5-14	14.69	15.88	17.63
5-15	14.88	16.06	17.81
6-0	15.0	16.19	18.0
6-1	15.19	16.38	18.19
6-2	15.31	16.56	18.38
6-3	15.5	16.69	18.56

(continues)

Table of Daily Breastmilk Volume Requirement Estimates (in Ounces)

BABY WEIGHT (LB-OZ)	REQUIRED MILK (2.5)	CATCH-UP MILK 1 (2.7)	CATCH-UP MILK 2 (3.0)
6-4	15.63	16.88	18.75
6-5	15.81	17.06	18.94
6-6	15.94	17.19	19.13
6-7	16.13	17.38	19.31
6-8	16.25	17.56	19.5
6-9	16.44	17.75	19.69
6-10	16.56	17.88	19.88
6-11	16.75	18.06	20.06
6-12	16.88	18.25	20.25
6-13	17.06	18.38	20.44
6-14	17.19	18.56	20.63
6-15	17.38	18.75	20.81
7-0	17.5	18.88	21.0
7-1	17.69	19.06	21.19
7-2	17.81	19.25	21.38
7-3	18.0	19.44	21.56
7-4	18.13	19.56	21.75
7-5	18.31	19.75	21.94
7-6	18.44	19.94	22.13
7-7	18.63	20.06	22.31
7-8	18.75	20.25	22.5
7-9	18.94	20.44	22.69
7-10	19.06	20.56	22.88

Table of Daily Breastmilk Volume Requirement Estimates (in Ounces)

BABY WEIGHT (LB-OZ)	REQUIRED MILK (2.5)	CATCH-UP MILK 1 (2.7)	CATCH-UP MILK 2 (3.0)
7-11	19.25	20.75	23.06
7-12	19.38	20.94	23.25
7-13	19.56	21.13	23.44
7-14	19.69	21.25	23.63
7-15	19.88	21.44	23.81
8-0	20.0	21.63	24.0
8-1	20.19	21.75	24.19
8-2	20.31	21.94	24.38
8-3	20.5	22.13	24.56
8-4	20.63	22.25	24.75
8-5	20.81	22.44	24.94
8-6	20.94	22.63	25.13
8-7	21.13	22.81	25.31
8-8	21.25	22.94	25.5
8-9	21.44	23.13	25.69
8-10	21.56	23.31	25.88
8-11	21.75	23.44	26.06
8-12	21.88	23.63	26.25
8-13	22.06	23.81	26.44
8-14	22.19	23.94	26.63
8-15	22.38	24.13	26.81
9-0	22.5	24.31	27.0

(continues)

APPENDICES

Table of Daily Breastmilk Volume Requirement Estimates (in Ounces)

BABY WEIGHT (LB-OZ)	REQUIRED MILK (2.5)	CATCH-UP MILK 1 (2.7)	CATCH-UP MILK 2 (3.0)
9-1	22.69	24.5	27.19
9-2	22.81	24.63	27.38
9-3	23.0	24.81	27.56
9-4	23.13	25.0	27.75
9-5	23.31	25.06	27.94
9-6	23.44	25.31	28.13
9-7	23.63	25.5	28.31
9-8	23.75	25.63	28.5
9-9	23.95	25.81	28.69
9-10	24.06	26.0	28.88
9-11	24.25	26.19	29.06
9-12	24.38	26.31	29.25
9-13	24.56	26.5	29.44
9-14	24.69	26.69	29.63
9-15	24.88	26.81	29.81
10-0	25.0	27.0	30.0
10-1	25.19	27.19	30.19
10-2	25.31	27.31	30.38
10-3	25.5	27.5	30.56
10-4	25.63	27.69	30.75
10-5	25.81	27.88	30.94
10-6	25.94	28.0	31.13

Table of Daily Breastmilk Volume Requirement Estimates (in Ounces)

BABY WEIGHT (LB-OZ)	REQUIRED MILK (2.5)	CATCH-UP MILK 1 (2.7)	CATCH-UP MILK 2 (3.0)
10-7	26.13	28.19	31.31
10-8	26.25	28.38	31.5
10-9	26.44	28.5	31.69
10-10	26.56	28.69	31.88
10-11	26.75	28.88	32.06
10-12	26.88	29.0	32.25
10-13	27.06	29.19	32.44
10-14	27.19	29.38	32.63
10-15	27.38	29.56	32.81

APPENDICES

APPENDIX G-2

Table of Daily Breastmilk Volume Requirement Estimates (in Grams and Milliliters)

BABY WEIGHT (GRAMS)	REQUIRED MILK (MILLILITERS)	CATCH-UP MILK 1 (MILLILITERS)	CATCH-UP MILK 2 (MILLILITERS)
2,000	330	360	400
2,050	340	370	410
2,100	350	380	420
2,150	360	380	430
2,200	360	390	440
2,250	370	400	450
2,300	380	410	460
2,350	390	420	470
2,400	400	430	480
2,450	410	440	490
2,500	410	450	500
2,550	420	460	510
2,600	430	460	520
2,650	440	470	530
2,700	450	480	540
2,750	460	490	550
2,800	460	500	560
2,850	470	510	570
2,900	480	520	580
2,950	490	530	590

Table of Daily Breastmilk Volume Requirement Estimates (in Grams and Milliliters)

BABY WEIGHT (GRAMS)	REQUIRED MILK (MILLILITERS)	CATCH-UP MILK 1 (MILLILITERS)	CATCH-UP MILK 2 (MILLILITERS)
3,000	500	540	600
3,050	500	550	610
3,100	510	550	620
3,150	520	560	630
3,200	530	570	640
3,250	540	580	650
3,300	550	590	660
3,350	550	600	670
3,400	560	610	680
3,450	570	620	690
3,500	580	630	700
3,550	590	630	710
3,600	600	640	720
3,650	600	650	730
3,700	610	660	740
3,750	620	670	750
3,800	630	680	750
3,850	640	690	760
3,900	650	700	770
3,950	650	710	780
4,000	660	720	790

(continues)

Table of Daily Breastmilk Volume Requirement Estimates (in Grams and Milliliters)

BABY WEIGHT (GRAMS)	REQUIRED MILK (MILLILITERS)	CATCH-UP MILK 1 (MILLILITERS)	CATCH-UP MILK 2 (MILLILITERS)
4,050	670	720	800
4,100	680	730	810
4,150	690	740	820
4,200	700	750	830
4,250	700	760	840
4,300	710	770	850
4,350	720	780	860
4,400	730	790	870
4,450	740	800	880
4,500	750	800	890
4,550	750	810	900
4,600	760	820	910
4,650	770	830	920
4,700	780	840	930
4,750	790	850	940
4,800	790	860	950
4,850	800	870	960
4,900	810	880	970
4,950	820	890	980
5,000	830	890	990

APPENDIX H-1

Baby Weight Loss Table (LB-OZ)

BIRTH WEIGHT (LB-OZ)	5% WEIGHT LOSS (LB-OZ)	7% WEIGHT LOSS (LB-OZ)	10% WEIGHT LOSS (LB-OZ)
5-0	4-12	4-10	4-8
5-1	4-13	4-11	4-9
5-2	4-14	4-12	4-10
5-3	4-15	4-13	4-11
5-4	4-15	4-14	4-12
5-5	5-1	4-15	4-13
5-6	5-2	5-0	4-13
5-7	5-3	5-1	4-14
5-8	5-4	5-2	4-15
5-9	5-5	5-3	5-0
5-10	5-6	5-4	5-1
5-11	5-6	5-5	5-2
5-12	5-7	5-6	5-3
5-13	5-8	5-6	5-4
5-14	5-9	5-7	5-5
5-15	5-10	5-8	5-6
6-0	5-11	5-9	5-6
6-1	5-12	5-10	5-7
6-2	5-13	5-11	5-8
6-3	5-14	5-12	5-9

(continues)

Baby Weight Loss Table (LB-OZ)

BIRTH WEIGHT (LB-OZ)	5% WEIGHT LOSS (LB-OZ)	7% WEIGHT LOSS (LB-OZ)	10% WEIGHT LOSS (LB-OZ)
6-4	5-15	5-13	5-10
6-5	6-0	5-14	5-11
6-6	6-1	5-15	5-12
6-7	6-2	6-0	5-13
6-8	6-3	6-1	5-14
6-9	6-4	6-2	5-15
6-10	6-5	6-3	5-15
6-11	6-6	6-4	6-0
6-12	6-7	6-4	6-1
6-13	6-8	6-5	6-2
6-14	6-9	6-6	6-3
6-15	6-9	6-7	6-4
7-0	6-10	6-8	6-5
7-1	6-11	6-9	6-6
7-2	6-12	6-10	6-7
7-3	6-13	6-11	6-8
7-4	6-14	6-12	6-8
7-5	6-15	6-13	6-9
7-6	7-0	6-14	6-10
7-7	7-1	6-15	6-11
7-8	7-2	7-0	6-12
7-9	7-3	7-1	6-13
7-10	7-4	7-1	6-14

Baby Weight Loss Table (LB-OZ)

BIRTH WEIGHT (LB-OZ)	5% WEIGHT LOSS (LB-OZ)	7% WEIGHT LOSS (LB-OZ)	10% WEIGHT LOSS (LB-OZ)
7-11	7-5	7-2	6-15
7-12	7-6	7-3	7-0
7-13	7-7	7-4	7-1
7-14	7-8	7-5	7-1
7-15	7-9	7-6	7-2
8-0	7-10	7-7	7-3
8-1	7-11	7-8	7-4
8-2	7-12	7-9	7-5
8-3	7-12	7-10	7-6
8-4	7-13	7-11	7-7
8-5	7-14	7-12	7-8
8-6	7-15	7-13	7-9
8-7	8-0	7-14	7-10
8-8	8-1	7-14	7-10
8-9	8-2	7-15	7-11
8-10	8-3	8-0	7-12
8-11	8-4	8-1	7-13
8-12	8-5	8-2	7-14
8-13	8-6	8-3	7-15
8-14	8-7	8-4	8-0
8-15	8-8	8-5	8-1
9-0	8-9	8-6	8-2

(continues)

APPENDICES

Baby Weight Loss Table (LB-OZ)

BIRTH WEIGHT (LB-OZ)	5% WEIGHT LOSS (LB-OZ)	7% WEIGHT LOSS (LB-OZ)	10% WEIGHT LOSS (LB-OZ)
9-1	8-10	8-7	8-3
9-2	8-11	8-8	8-3
9-3	8-12	8-9	8-4
9-4	8-13	8-10	8-5
9-5	8-14	8-11	8-6
9-6	8-15	8-12	8-7
9-7	8-15	8-12	8-8
9-8	9-0	8-13	8-9
9-9	9-1	8-14	8-10
9-10	9-2	8-15	8-11
9-11	9-3	9-0	8-12
9-12	9-4	9-1	8-12
9-13	9-5	9-2	8-13
9-14	9-6	9-3	8-14
9-15	9-7	9-4	8-15
10-0	9-8	9-5	9-0
10-1	9-9	9-6	9-1
10-2	9-10	9-7	9-2
10-3	9-11	9-8	9-3
10-4	9-12	9-9	9-4
10-5	9-13	9-9	9-5
10-6	9-14	9-10	9-5
10-7	9-15	9-11	9-6

Baby Weight Loss Table (LB-OZ)

BIRTH WEIGHT (LB-OZ)	5% WEIGHT LOSS (LB-OZ)	7% WEIGHT LOSS (LB-OZ)	10% WEIGHT LOSS (LB-OZ)
10-8	10-0	9-12	9-7
10-9	10-1	9-13	9-8
10-10	10-2	9-14	9-9
10-11	10-2	9-15	9-10
10-12	10-3	10-0	9-11
10-13	10-4	10-1	9-12
10-14	10-5	10-2	9-13
10-15	10-6	10-3	9-14

APPENDIX H-2

Baby Weight Loss Table (Grams)

BIRTH WEIGHT (GRAMS)	5% WEIGHT LOSS (GRAMS)	7% WEIGHT LOSS (GRAMS)	10% WEIGHT LOSS (GRAMS)
2,000	1,900	1,860	1,800
2,050	1,947.5	1,906.5	1,845
2,100	1,995	1,953	1,890
2,150	2,042.5	1,999.5	1,935
2,200	2,090	2,046	1,980
2,250	2,137.5	2,092.5	2,025
2,300	2,185	2,139	2,070
2,350	2,232.5	2,185.5	2,115
2,400	2,280	2,232	2,160
2,450	2,327.5	2,278.5	2,205
2,500	2,375	2,325	2,250
2,550	2,422.5	2,371.5	2,295
2,600	2,470	2,418	2,340
2,650	2,517.5	2,464.5	2,385
2,700	2,565	2,511	2,430
2,750	2,612.5	2,557.5	2,475
2,800	2,660	2,604	2,520
2,850	2,707.5	2,650.5	2,565
2,900	2,755	2,697	2,610
2,950	2,802.5	2,743.5	2,655
3,000	2,850	2,790	2,700

Baby Weight Loss Table (Grams)

Birth Weight (grams)	5% Weight Loss (grams)	7% Weight Loss (grams)	10% Weight Loss (grams)
3,050	2,897.5	2,836.5	2,745
3,100	2,945	2,883	2,790
3,150	2,992.5	2,929.5	2,835
3,200	3,040	2,976	2,880
3,250	3,087.5	3,022.5	2,925
3,300	3,135	3,069	2,970
3,350	3,182.5	3,115.5	3,015
3,400	3,230	3,162	3,060
3,450	3,277.5	3,208.5	3,105
3,500	3,325	3,255	3,150
3,550	3,372.5	3,301.5	3,195
3,600	3,420	3,348	3,240
3,650	3,467.5	3,394.5	3,285
3,700	3,515	3,441	3,330
3,750	3,562.5	3,487.5	3,375
3,800	3,610	3,534	3,420
3,850	3,657.5	3,580.5	3,465
3,900	3,705	3,627	3,510
3,950	3,752.5	3,673.5	3,555
4,000	3,800	3,720	3,600
4,050	3,847.5	3,766.5	3,645
4,100	3,895	3,813	3,690

APPENDICES

(continues)

Baby Weight Loss Table (Grams)

Birth Weight (Grams)	5% Weight Loss (Grams)	7% Weight Loss (Grams)	10% Weight Loss (Grams)
4,150	3,942.5	3,859.5	3,735
4,200	3,990	3,906	3,780
4,250	4,037.5	3,952.5	3,825
4,300	4,085	3,999	3,870
4,350	4,132.5	4,045.5	3,915
4,400	4,180	4,092	3,960
4,450	4,227.5	4,138.5	4,005
4,500	4,275	4,185	4,050
4,550	4,322.5	4,231.5	4,095
4,600	4,370	4,278	4,140
4,650	4,417.5	4,324.5	4,185
4,700	4,465	4,371	4,230
4,750	4,512.5	4,417.5	4,275
4,800	4,560	4,464	4,320
4,850	4,607.5	4,510.5	4,365
4,900	4,655	4,557	4,410
4,950	4,702.5	4,603.5	4,455
5,000	4,750	4,650	4,500

APPENDIX I

Weight Gain Expectations and Infant Elimination Patterns

According to the AAP Section on Breastfeeding (2012, p. e835):

> All breastfeeding newborn infants should be seen by a pediatrician at 3 to 5 days of age, which is within 48 to 72 hours after discharge from the hospital:
>
> - Evaluate hydration (elimination patterns).
> - Evaluate body weight gain (body weight loss no more than 7 percent from birth and no further weight loss by day 5: assess feeding and consider more frequent follow-up).
> - Discuss maternal/infant issues.
> - Observe feeding.

At the Center for Breastfeeding, we expect a baby to have four stools (some yellow) daily by day 4. We also expect the baby to be back at birth weight by 12 to 14 days of age. If not, an intensive in-person evaluation of breastfeeding, milk supply, and milk transfer with corrective interventions is initiated.

In the early months, we expect, at a minimum, a weight gain of approximately 1 ounce per day, although our observation is that most healthy breastfed babies gain more than an ounce a day, on average.

APPENDIX J

Protocol for Building a Milk Supply/Relactation

Virtually every woman can produce enough milk for her baby. If a mother has a low milk supply, she may want to increase the amount of milk she is making. The following protocol is the one we use at the Center for Breastfeeding for low milk supply.

Determine the reason for low supply:

Low milk supply can result if:

- Breastfeeding gets off to a suboptimal start (not breastfeeding frequently enough; pumping for weeks for a premie; overuse of a pacifier).
- The mother chooses not to breastfeed and then later changes her mind.
- The mother has been smoking cigarettes.
- The mother has taken certain medications, including decongestants containing pseudoephedrine.
- The mother has physiological problems that are the underlying cause for poor milk supply, such as:
  - Inadequate breast tissue.
  - Class 3 inverted nipples.
  - Postpartum hemorrhage (with resulting pituitary insult).
  - Breast surgery/injury.
  - Abnormal levels of thyroid hormones (if/when these are corrected, milk supply can rebound).
  - Retained placental fragment(s).

Consider the potential for altering the conditions that contributed to the condition of poor/low/no milk supply:

A realistic assessment of the reason for the low milk supply should precede the planning phase:

- If the mother was nursing on a schedule only six times a day or had hypothyroidism (now normal due to medication), plan to build the supply and increase the transfer of milk to the baby.
- If the mother has a nonmodifiable or only partially modifiable issue such as inadequate breast tissue, profound breast reduction surgery, or class 3 inverted nipples, it may be physiologically impossible to increase her milk supply to meet the baby's total needs.

Determine the mother's goals:

Is her goal:

- To exclusively breastfeed at the breast?
- To provide her milk via a supplemental feeding method?
- To breastfeed and supplement with formula?

Assess the current milk supply/transfer:

By estimating how much milk is currently available by expression or transfer to the baby, it will be possible to monitor increase.

- If the mother is expressing milk only, ask the mother to log the volumes of as many expressions as possible.
- If the mother is breastfeeding, estimate milk transfer using the protocol in Appendix E.

Estimate the baby's daily needs (Appendix F), and determine how much the mother needs to express or transfer to the baby while nursing:

Estimate the amount the mother is expressing/transferring, and subtract that from the amount the baby needs. Here's an example:

- The baby was born at 6 pounds and was not very active when nursing. The mother fed every 3 to 4 hours, and the baby weighs 5 pounds 11 ounces at 2 weeks.
- She has no other known risks for low milk supply.
- The pediatric care provider has determined that the baby needs to "catch up," meaning a need for 15.6 to 17.1 ounces per day.
- The mother tells us that she is only feeding the baby at the breast. She nurses eight times a day.
- When we do pre- and postfeeding weights, we see that the baby transfers 0.5 ounce on one breast and 1 ounce on the other. If this is typical, then the baby is receiving:

$$1.5 \times 8 = 12 \text{ ounces}$$

- We estimate a need for milk volume to increase by 4 to 5 ounces a day. (Note: The pediatric care provider should take the lead in determining the estimated need.)

Determine how the baby is being fed now:
- Breast?
- Cup?
- Bottle?
- At-breast feeder?
- Other?

Consider available methods to increase milk supply:
- Is expression an available method of increasing milk collection/supply?
- Is the baby willing and able to nurse?
- Would the addition of an at-breast feeder increase breast stimulation and work to increase supply?

Consider the nature of and delivery method for additional milk:
- Is the baby being fed formula? Could it be replaced ounce for ounce with expressed milk?
- Is safe donor milk available to the mother? (See HMBANA in Appendix Y.)
- Which supplementation methods will suit this family and also protect the future of breastfeeding? (Appendix N)

Make a plan for monitoring and follow-up:
- At the Center for Breastfeeding, we would encourage the mother experiencing milk production problems to consider combining hand expression with pumping with a rental-grade, double-pumping system.
- We would work closely with the baby's pediatric care provider to monitor the baby's weight gain daily, and to negotiate use of expressed or donor human milk (as available) to replace formula.
- When the mother can express and feed a substantial amount (75 to 80 percent) of the amount that is needed to make up the deficit, we would again assess milk transfer (Appendix E).
- We might also consider having the mother weigh the baby in her home with a digital scale (accurate to 2 grams) to monitor the baby's

transfer. We often do this with premies who are discharged receiving half or more of the intake of formula so that the mother can more accurately determine how much formula to use as a supplement after breastfeeding.

- We would recalculate needs as the baby grows.

APPENDIX K

Protocol for Oversupply of Breastmilk

For many years, poor breastfeeding management practices highlighted the issue of "not enough breastmilk." In our experience, oversupply of breastmilk seems to be increasingly common as more and more mothers choose to breastfeed and breastfeed exclusively and for longer durations. It is also more likely to happen with the mother's second or subsequent breastfeeding babies.

Signs of oversupply:

- Nipple pain is worse after the first few days with an abundant supply of milk. (Sometimes a baby can manage the slower flow of colostrum but has trouble managing the abundant and rapid flow of milk after day 3 or 4.) The pain is related to the baby clamping down on the nipple because the flow of milk is too abundant or too rapid for the baby to handle.
- Baby gags, chokes, and/or coughs at the breast as if the milk is coming too fast.
- Baby spits up and is gassy after feedings.
- Baby pulls off the breast while nursing and milk sprays.
- Nipple is compressed or discolored at the end of the nursing.
- Mother experiences painful nipples, frequent plugged ducts, and/or episodes of mastitis.
- Baby gains weight rapidly, more than an ounce a day. (We have seen babies gaining more than a pound a week.)

- Baby has many large explosive bowel movements (comes out of diaper).
- Although the baby is gaining well, the baby may still not act contented between feedings, giving the mother the mistaken idea that she doesn't have enough milk or that there is something wrong with her milk.
- Weights taken before and after nursing with a digital scale accurate to 2 grams show rapid transfer of more than expected amounts of milk at the breast in a shorter than expected amount of time (for example, 4 ounces in 5 minutes).

What to do about it:

- Help the mother achieve a posture where the baby is able to move his or her head freely when the flow of milk is too great or fast to handle. One position that works well is where the mother is reclining or semi-reclining and the baby's body is supported on the mother's (Figure C-4). The mother is "down under" the baby (which is why it is called the Australian posture—see **Figure K-1**). The baby no longer has to work against the milk flow.

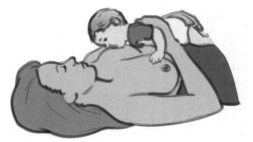

Courtesy of Healthy Children Project

Figure K-1 When using the Australian posture, the mother is "down under."

- More aggressive treatment may include nursing on only one breast at each feeding to allow a small amount of breast compression in order to tamp back the supply. (This technique is known as "block feeding.") A firm bra may also help. The mother must be careful not to allow too much pressure because doing so could foster mastitis. Encourage the mother to check her breasts daily for any red or swollen areas.
- In some cases, women have needed to nurse on one breast for two or more feedings in a row to decrease milk production. In these cases, encourage her to monitor the unsuckled breast closely for any signs of redness and swelling.
- We have had good success with mothers who expressed until their breasts were soft before starting block feeding. This should only be done once, as continued expression will perpetuate the overproduction of milk.
- Instead of decreasing the milk supply using compression, some mothers prefer to collect the extra milk and donate to a mothers' milk bank. Contact the Human Milk Banking Association for further information (Appendix Y).

APPENDICES

Expected resolution:
- Although there may be some residual pain for a day or so if the nipple has been damaged, the mother's pain level should disappear with the baby in control of the flow rather than feeding against it.
- The nipple should not be distorted after nursing.

What else to consider:
- Hand expression or pumping to get rid of the "extra" milk may compound the problem by relieving the compression on the cells. As a result, the milk supply continues to increase.

APPENDIX L

Improving Milk Transfer

Improving milk transfer should be part of a larger assessment process that includes pre- and postfeeding weights with a scale accurate to 2 grams. (See protocol in Appendix E.) Some corrective interventions for poor milk transfer are as follows:

- Scrupulously observe for feeding cues. Feed the baby at the baby's best time.
- Try different positions (cross-cradle, semi-reclining, football, upright) to determine if there is better transfer in one or the other (Appendix C).
- Some babies nurse better when their hips are flexed and feet are flat against the back of a chair or another surface, as in **Figure L-1**.
- Ensure that the baby's arms are free and able to encircle the breast.
- Ensure that the baby's body is in alignment— head over shoulders, shoulders over hips.
- Ensure that the baby is aligned nose to nipple to start.

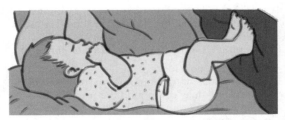

Courtesy of Healthy Children Project

Figure L-1 Baby's hips are flexed and feet are flat against a pillow.

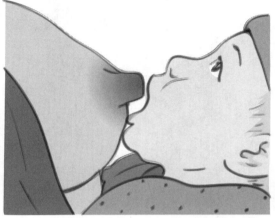

Courtesy of Healthy Children Project

Figure L-2 The baby's head tilts back and the mouth gapes. The lower lip and chin reach the breast first.

- Ensure that the mother's hand, finger, or arm is not putting pressure on the back of the baby's head.
- Ensure that the baby's head can tilt back, as in **Figure L-2**, to allow maximum jaw excursion and wide-open mouth, as in **Figure L-3**.
- If baby stops suckling and appears to go to sleep, ask the mother to use breast compression/ alternate massage to change the rate of flow of the milk. Observe for sucking and swallowing.
- Use alternate massage/breast compression (Appendix D) to move the milk. At each pause, suck, swallow, compress breast; suck, swallow, compress breast, as in **Figure L-4**.

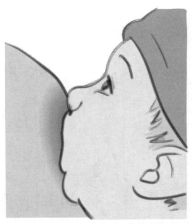

Courtesy of Healthy Children Project

Figure L-3 The baby is positioned asymmetrically at the breast.

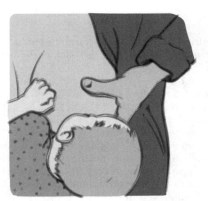

Courtesy of Healthy Children Project

Figure L-4 Alternate massage or breast compression is a way to increase the flow of milk to the baby. The mother compresses the breast when the baby pauses.

- Have the mother move the baby into a semi-upright position with flexed hips, as in **Figure L-5**. In this position, the baby may be more wakeful.
- Use expressed milk in an at-breast feeder.
- Consider the use of a nipple shield, combined with milk expression to protect the milk supply.
- Ensure continued monitoring of milk transfer.
- WARNING: Seek emergent medical care if any pediatric warning signs (Appendix Z) are observed or suspected. Occasionally, problems with inadequate milk transfer reflect a pediatric medical condition.

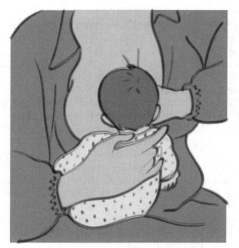

Courtesy of Healthy Children Project

Figure L-5 A premie, a baby with a cleft palate, or a neurologically challenged baby may nurse better in a more upright position.

APPENDIX M

Expression of Breastmilk

HAND EXPRESSION

Many women find that hand expression is easier and faster than using a mechanical breast pump. Another advantage to hand expression is that there is little to clean or get contaminated (e.g., tubing, gaskets).

How we teach hand expression:
- Wash your hands.
- Have a clean container ready to collect the milk. The newer you are to hand expression, the wider the container should be. Start with a large, lightweight bowl for the first few expressions.
- Do light breast massage right down to your nipples. Give them a little stretch to get the hormones flowing.
- Place your thumb and index finger on your areola, as in **Figure M-1**.
- Pull back toward your chest wall, then compress your thumb and finger together gently and rhythmically, mimicking the suckling of the baby (about one compression per second). It is best if you do not slide your fingers on your skin. Some women like to use a rolling motion.
- Position the collecting container on a table if you are standing up, or on your lap if you are sitting down. Try to aim the spray into the container.
- Repeat the motion of pulling back and compressing gently in the same place on your breast until the flow slows down.
- Move the finger and thumb to another spot and repeat.

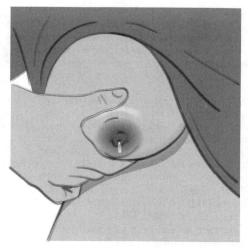

Courtesy of Healthy Children Project

Figure M-1 To hand express milk, the mother
positions her hand behind the areola and moves her
thumb and fingers together without sliding on the skin.
Many mothers find it effective to push back against
the chest wall before compressing the breast with the
thumb and finger.

- Switch to the other breast.
- Really proficient expressers can do both breasts
  simultaneously, but they usually need two
  containers!

BREAST PUMPS

- Breast pumps should always be used and cleaned
  according to the manufacturer's instructions.
  A list of pump company websites and other
  information may be found in Appendix Y.

- Combining hand expression with pumping is a good way to maximize milk yield (Flaherman et al., 2012; Morton et al., 2009).
- There is no pump that is right for every mother and every situation. Some pumps are better for pump-dependent mothers and some are better for occasional use.
- Any pump can cause damage when used incorrectly.
- The U.S. Food and Drug Administration (FDA) maintains a database of pump complaints in the Manufacturer and User Facility Device Experience Database (MAUDE). See Appendix Y for more information. It is wise to check the database before considering pumps. Also, injuries related to breast pump use should be reported to the MAUDE site.
- There are several things to consider about operating a breast pump, such as whether it is powered by personal energy (for example, hand or foot powered) or powered by electricity, or whether it pumps one breast at a time or both together.
- Do not use parts from one company on another company's pumps.

In Our Opinion

An important consideration is whether the pump is a personal pump (single-user pump) or multi-user pump. Single user means that once the pump is used by one person, the manufacturer does not warrant that the pump itself can be cleaned sufficiently (even if new tubing, bottles, etc., were used) for the safety of a second mother and baby to be exposed to it. The FDA (2013) has a strong statement regarding used breastpumps:

> Only breast pumps that are designed for multiple users should be used by more than

one person. With the exception of multiple user pumps, the FDA considers breast pumps to be single-user devices. That means that a breast pump should only be used by one woman because there is no way to guarantee the pump can be cleaned and disinfected between uses by different women.

Breast pumps that are reused by different mothers can carry infectious particles, which can make you or your baby sick.

Buying a used breast pump or sharing a breast pump may be a violation of the manufacturer's warranty and you may not be able to get help from the manufacturer if you have a problem with the pump.

This means that it is up to the manufacturer to decide whether or not the pump is single or multiple use. Always check with the manufacturer (not the store or other vendor) about whether a pump is approved for a second user, which parts need to be replaced before a second mother uses the pump, and what cleaning methods and products should be used.

We can't stress caution enough! Pumps bought at yard sales, bought on the Internet, or borrowed from a friend can transmit diseases from one mother to another mother's baby!

APPENDIX N

Feeding Devices

AT-BREAST FEEDERS
- Baby gets additional milk while at the breast through a tube attached to a reservoir.
- Mother's body gets the message to make more milk while baby is getting additional milk from the supplemental feeding device.
- Sources are listed in Appendix Y.
- Hospitals often use syringes with feeding tubes attached.

CUP FEEDING
- Cups are inexpensive, available, and easy to clean.
- A growing body of research indicates the safety and efficacy for both term and preterm infants.
- Baby sets his or her own pace.
- When cup feeding, sit the baby upright. Do not pour the milk into the baby's mouth. Tip the cup slightly so that the milk is at the edge of the cup. Rest the cup gently on the baby's lower lip. The baby may sip, slurp, or lap milk from the cup.

SPOON FEEDING
- We like to use small plastic spoons to collect drops of expressed colostrum if needed for the first few days.
- Coach parents to use the spoon to dribble a drop or two of milk on the baby's lips. If in the right state for feeding, the baby is likely to lap or lick milk from the spoon. Even small amounts of colostrum or human milk delivered via the spoon are enough to spur baby's interest and energy.

APPENDIX O

What to Do If an Infant or Child Is Mistakenly Fed Another Woman's Expressed Breastmilk

This section is extracted from the U.S. Centers for Disease Control and Prevention (2009b):

If a child has been mistakenly fed another child's bottle of expressed breast milk, the possible exposure to HIV or other infectious diseases should be treated just as if an accidental exposure to other body fluids had occurred.

The provider should:

1. Inform the mother who expressed the breast milk of the bottle switch, and ask
   ○ When the breast milk was expressed and how it was handled prior to being delivered to the caretaker or facility.
   ○ Whether she has ever had an HIV test and, if so, would she be willing to share the results with the parents of the child given the incorrect milk?
   ○ If she does not know whether she has ever been tested for HIV, would she be willing to contact her physician and find out if she has been tested?
   ○ If she has never been tested for HIV, would she be willing to have one and share the results with the parents of the other child?
2. Discuss the mistaken milk with the parents of the child who was given the wrong bottle.
   ○ Inform them that their child was given another child's bottle of expressed breast milk.

- ○ Inform them that the risk of transmission of HIV is very small.
- ○ Encourage the parents to notify the child's physician of the exposure.
- ○ Provide the family with information on when the milk was expressed and how the milk was handled prior to its being delivered to the caretaker so that the parents may inform their own physician.
- ○ Inform the parents that their child should soon undergo a baseline test for HIV.

The risk of HIV transmission from expressed breast milk consumed by another child is believed to be low because

- In the United States, women who are HIV positive, and aware of that fact, are advised NOT to breastfeed their infants.
- Chemicals present in breast milk, act together with time and cold temperatures, to destroy the HIV present in expressed breast milk.
- Transmission of HIV from single breast milk exposure has never been documented.

APPENDIX P
Handling and Storing Breastmilk

Breastmilk is a raw food, and even though it is teeming with antibodies and other protective elements, care should be taken in the collection, handling, and storage processes. Everything that comes into contact with milk should be clean and dry. If the baby is premature, fragile, ill, or hospitalized, there may be additional precautions recommended by the hospital or caregivers. For example, certain containers may be specified, and the containers must be sterilized, not merely clean. In some cases, milk for hospitalized babies may need to be frozen right away or never frozen.

Breastmilk Storage Containers

Reusable glass or plastic, hard-sided containers are considered the best for storing breastmilk. It is important that the cap fits securely. The same companies that make pumps and other equipment make milk storage containers. In addition, some companies make hard-sided containers specifically for breastmilk (Appendix Y). Other hard-sided plastic food storage containers with tight lids as well as small glass jars may also be used.

Plastic bags are also available that have been specifically manufactured to collect and store mother's milk. Some of these fit into the container that milk is pumped into in pumping systems, and the bags also may fit into baby feeding bottles. Bags can be easily contaminated during handling; they are awkward to handle and can also leak.

Each container of milk should be labeled, at a minimum, with the date. When a baby is premature or hospitalized for any reason, the hospital will either give the mother labels for her milk or provide her with specific information that should be on the label including date, patient ID number, unit, and so on. If the milk will be going to a day-care setting, the baby's name should be clearly legible and written with a waterproof, smudge-proof marker.

In Our Opinion

If a mother is going to store a lot of milk, we would encourage her to try samples of a few different storage systems before she invests in one.

If a mother chooses to freeze milk in bags, we would encourage her to put a group of them inside a freezer-grade plastic bag.

STORING MILK

Individualized storage recommendations will be given to the mother if the milk is being stored for a premature, fragile, ill, or hospitalized baby. Some neonatal intensive care units use only frozen milk; in other cases, the milk should not be frozen or warmed so as to preserve all of the components of human milk. If the baby is hospitalized, the instructions may include storing and freezing the milk in the same small quantities that the baby is being fed.

How long can milk be kept at room temperature, in the refrigerator, or in the freezer?

We asked our colleague, Lois Arnold, PhD, this question, and she developed the algorithm in **Figure P-1**. You may notice that her suggestions are more conservative than some others you may see; that's because they are public health recommendations based on the evidence and aimed at keeping milk at the highest possible quality.

To use this algorithm, ask the mother when she will need the milk.

- You can safely store milk for 3 to 5 days in the refrigerator. However, put it in the freezer as soon as you can if you are going to freeze it.

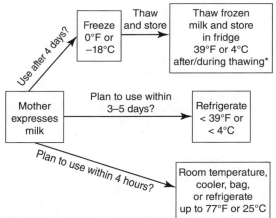

*Do not microwave human milk

Courtesy of Lois Arnold, PhD, MPH, ALC of the American Breastfeeding Institute.

Figure P-1 Public health recommendations for safe storage of breastmilk for healthy term babies.

- Milk may be kept up to 3 months in a refrigerator freezer and 6 months in a deep freeze that is kept at −20°F or less.
- Over the course of a day, small expressions of chilled milk can be added to milk stored in the refrigerator.
- Always place the milk in the coldest part of the refrigerator or freezer. That is usually not on the door or near the fan in a frost-free type of freezer.

THAWING AND WARMING BREASTMILK

- Always thaw frozen breastmilk in the container in which it was frozen.
- The refrigerator is an excellent place to defrost frozen milk.
- Refrigerated or frozen milk can be warmed in a pan of lukewarm water or under lukewarm, running tap water.
- Never use a microwave to thaw or warm breastmilk or any other baby foods. There are cases in which babies have been burned because "hot spots" were not detectable by the adult. Breastmilk is especially vulnerable to microwaves, and components can be damaged.
- Thawed breastmilk should be kept cold until just before being fed to the baby.
- Thawed breastmilk should be used within 24 hours of being defrosted.
- Thawed breastmilk should not be refrozen.

In Our Opinion

Milk should be stored in containers in the amount that the baby is going to be offered at one feeding, not stored in the amount that the mother has expressed. Expressed mother's milk is a valuable commodity that deserves careful handling.

APPENDIX Q

Contraindications to Breastfeeding

This section is extracted from the Centers for Disease Control and Prevention website (2015).

WHEN SHOULD A MOTHER AVOID BREASTFEEDING?

Health professionals agree that human milk provides the most complete form of nutrition for infants, including premature and sick newborns. However, there are rare exceptions when human milk is not recommended. Under certain circumstances, a physician will need to make a case-by-case assessment to determine whether a woman's environmental exposure or her own medical condition warrants her to interrupt or stop breastfeeding.

Breastfeeding is NOT advisable if one or more of the following conditions is true:

1. An infant diagnosed with galactosemia, a rare genetic metabolic disorder
2. The infant whose mother:
   - Has been infected with the human immunodeficiency virus (HIV).
   - Is taking antiretroviral medications.
   - Has untreated, active tuberculosis.
   - Is infected with human T-cell lymphotropic virus type I or type II.
   - Is using or is dependent upon an illicit drug.
   - Is taking prescribed cancer chemotherapy agents, such as antimetabolites, that interfere with DNA replication and cell division.

○ Is undergoing radiation therapies; however, such nuclear medicine therapies require only a temporary interruption in breastfeeding.

In Our Opinion

Other lists of contraindicated conditions exist (WHO, 2009; AAP, 2012). For example, in addition to the issues identified above, AAP (2012) lists untreated brucellosis in the mother as a contraindication to breastfeeding. We think it is important that everyone in a given facility, agency, or system agree on which national or international contraindications list they are following and disseminate that information widely to all care providers.

APPENDIX R

Breastfeeding Goals for
the United States

According to the U.S. Department of Health and Human Services (2010), Healthy People 2020 is a set of goals and objectives with 10-year targets designed to guide national health promotion and disease prevention efforts to improve the health of all people in the United States. Released by the U.S. Department of Health and Human Services each decade, Healthy People reflects the idea that setting objectives and providing science-based benchmarks to track and monitor progress can motivate and focus action. Healthy People 2020 represents the fourth generation of this initiative, building on a foundation of three decades of work.

Since their inception in the late 1970s for the year 1990, the Healthy People goals have included breastfeeding targets. For the first time, the 2020 goals include targeted improvements in maternity care practices and workplace support.

The objectives for the Healthy People 2020 goals for breastfeeding at different time periods are found in **Table R-1**.

Note: These goals are up to date as of the publication date of this book. Midterm updates to the goals may be made in 2015, and new goals will be developed in 2020 for 2030. Visit the Healthy People website (Appendix Y) for updates.

243

Table R-1   Healthy People Goals

GOAL	2010 TARGET %	2014 CDC REPORT CARD %	2020 GOAL %
↑ Ever breastfed	75	79.2	81.9
↑ Breastfed at 6 months	50	49.4	60.6
↑ Breastfed at 12 months	25	26.7	34.1
↑ Exclusive at 3 months	40	40.7	46.2
↑ Exclusive at 6 months	17	18.8	25.5
↑ Workplace lactation support			38.0
↓ Formula use in the first 2 days		19.4	14.2
↑ Births in Baby-Friendly® designated facilities		7.79	8.1

APPENDIX S

Edinburgh Postnatal Depression Scale

The Edinburgh Postnatal Depression Scale [EPDS] was developed for screening postpartum women in outpatient, home visiting settings, or at the 6–8 week postpartum examination. It has been utilized among numerous populations including U.S. women and Spanish-speaking women in other countries. The EPDS consists of 10 questions. The test can usually be completed in less than 5 minutes.

Women should be asked to *rate their responses according to how they have felt in the past week*. Responses are scored 0, 1, 2, or 3 according to increased severity of the symptom. Items marked with an asterisk (*) are reverse scored (3, 2, 1, and 0). The total score is determined by adding together the scores for each of the 10 items. Validation studies have utilized various threshold scores in which women were positive and in need of referral. Cut-off scores ranged from 10 to 13 points.

Therefore, to err on safety's side, a woman scoring 10 or more points or indicating any suicidal ideation—that is, she scores 1 or higher on question #10—should be referred immediately for follow-up. Even if a woman scores 9 or lower, if the care provider feels she is suffering from depression, an appropriate referral should be made.

The EPDS is only a screening tool. It does not diagnose depression. High scores indicate that the mother should be referred to an appropriately licensed healthcare personnel, although the tool may be administered by any caregiver. Users may reproduce the scale without permission providing the copyright is respected by quoting the names of the authors, title, and the source of the paper in all reproduced copies.

INSTRUCTIONS FOR USERS

1. The mother is asked to underline 1 of 4 possible responses that comes the closest to how she has been feeling the previous 7 days.
2. All 10 items must be completed.
3. Care should be taken to avoid the possibility of the mother discussing her answers with others.
4. The mother should complete the scale herself, unless she has limited English or has difficulty with reading.

Name: _____
Date: _____
Address: _____
Baby's Age: _____

As you have recently had a baby, we would like to know how you are feeling. Please <u>underline</u> the answer that comes closest to how you have felt in the past 7 days, not just how you feel today.

Here is an example, already completed:
I have felt happy:
    Yes, all the time
    <u>Yes, most of the time</u>
    No, not very often
    No, not at all
This would mean: "I have felt happy most of the time" during the past week. Please complete the other questions in the same way.

In the past 7 days:

1. I have been able to laugh and see the funny side of things:
   As much as I always could
   Not quite so much now
   Definitely not so much now
   Not at all

2. I have looked forward with enjoyment to things:
   As much as I ever did
   Rather less than I used to
   Definitely less than I used to
   Hardly at all

*3. I have blamed myself unnecessarily when things went wrong:
   Yes, most of the time
   Yes, some of the time
   Not very often
   No, never

4. I have been anxious or worried for no good reason:
   No, not at all
   Hardly ever
   Yes, sometimes
   Yes, very often

*5. I have felt scared or panicky for no very good reason:
   Yes, quite a lot
   Yes, sometimes
   No, not much
   No, not at all

*6. Things have been getting on top of me:
   Yes, most of the time I haven't been able to cope at all.
   Yes, sometimes I haven't been coping as well as usual.
   No, most of the time I have coped quite well.
   No, I have been coping as well as ever.

*7. I have been so unhappy that I have had difficulty sleeping:

Yes, most of the time
Yes, sometimes
Not very often
No, not at all

*8. I have felt sad or miserable:
Yes, most of the time
Yes, quite often
Not very often
No, not at all

*9. I have been so unhappy that I have been crying:
Yes, most of the time
Yes, quite often
Only occasionally
No, never

*10. The thought of harming myself has occurred to me:
Yes, quite often
Sometimes
Hardly ever
Never

APPENDIX T

The International Code of Marketing of Breast-milk Substitutes (WHO, 1981)

Adopted in 1981 by the World Health Assembly, the International Code of Marketing of Breast-milk Substitutes is intended to protect and promote breastfeeding, through the provision of adequate information on appropriate infant feeding and the regulation of the marketing of breastmilk substitutes, bottles, and teats. In subsequent years, additional resolutions have further defined and strengthened the Code. According to the World Health Organization, UNICEF, and IBFAN (2016), 39 countries have adopted all or most of the Code's provisions as legislation or other legal measures. Thirty-one countries have adopted many provisions of the Code. Sixty-five countries have taken steps to adopt a few provisions. This means that 135 countries have had some legal or legislative action on the Code. Forty-nine countries, including the United States, have reported no legal or legislative measures in place. Information was not available for 10 additional countries.

According to UNICEF (2007), "The Code prohibits the advertisement or promotion of these products to the general public or through the health care system. All governments should adopt the Code into national legislation."

The International Code includes the following stipulations (UNICEF, 2007):

- "That neither health facilities nor health professionals should have a role in promoting breast-milk substitutes.
- That free samples should not be provided to pregnant women, new mothers, or families."

The text of the entire code may be found on the WHO website (Appendix Y).

APPENDIX U

The Global Strategy for Infant and Young Child Feeding (WHO, 2003)

The Global Strategy for Infant and Young Child Feeding is an initiative of the WHO and the United Nations Childrens' Fund (UNICEF) to build upon successful prior initiatives, especially the Innocenti Declaration and the Baby-Friendly Hospital Initiative. The Global Strategy includes the needs of all children, including those living in difficult circumstances such as infants of mothers living with HIV, low birth weight infants, and infants in emergency situations. The entire document may be found on the WHO's website (Appendix Y).

OPERATIONAL TARGETS

Four operational targets from the 1990 Innocenti Declaration (WHO & UNICEF, 1990):

1. Appoint a national breastfeeding coordinator with appropriate authority, and establish a multisectoral national breastfeeding committee composed of representatives from relevant government departments, nongovernmental organizations, and health professional associations.
2. Ensure that every facility providing maternity services fully follows all the "Ten steps to successful breastfeeding" set out in the WHO/UNICEF statement on breastfeeding and maternity services.

3. Give effect to the principles and aim of the International Code of Marketing of Breast-milk Substitutes and subsequent relevant Health Assembly resolutions in their entirety.

4. Enact imaginative legislation protecting the breastfeeding rights of working women and establish means for its enforcement.

Five additional operational targets:

5. Develop, implement, monitor, and evaluate a comprehensive policy on infant and young child feeding, in the context of national policies and programs for nutrition, child and reproductive health, and poverty reduction.

6. Ensure that the health and other relevant sectors protect, promote, and support exclusive breastfeeding for 6 months and continued breastfeeding up to 2 years of age or beyond, while providing women access to the support they require—in the family, community, and workplace—to achieve this goal.

7. Promote timely, adequate, safe, and appropriate complementary feeding with continued breastfeeding.

8. Provide guidance on feeding infants and young children in exceptionally difficult circumstances, and on the related support required by mothers, families, and other caregivers.

9. Consider what new legislation or other suitable measures may be required, as part of a comprehensive policy on infant and young child feeding, to give effect to the principles and aim of the International Code of Marketing of Breast-milk Substitutes and to subsequent relevant Health Assembly resolutions.

APPENDIX V

Innocenti Declaration on Infant and Young Child Feeding 2005 (WHO & UNICEF, 2005)

In the 15 years since the adoption of the original Innocenti Declaration in 1990, remarkable progress has been made in improving infant and young child feeding practices worldwide. Nevertheless, inappropriate feeding practices—suboptimal or no breastfeeding and inadequate complementary feeding—remain the greatest threat to child health and survival globally.

Improved breastfeeding alone could save the lives of more than 3,500 children every day, more than any other preventive intervention.

Guided by accepted human rights principles, especially those embodied in the Convention on the Rights of the Child, our vision is of an environment that enables mothers, families, and other caregivers to make informed decisions about optimal feeding, which is defined as exclusive breastfeeding for 6 months, followed by the introduction of appropriate complementary feeding and continuation of breastfeeding for up to 2 years of age or beyond.

Achieving this vision requires skilled practical support to arrive at the highest attainable standard of health and development for infants and young children, which is the universal right of every child.

Challenges remain: poverty, the HIV pandemic, natural and human-made emergencies, globalization, environmental contamination, health systems investing primarily in curative rather than preventive services, gender inequities, and women's increasing rates of employment outside the home, including in the nonformal sector. These challenges must be addressed to achieve the Millennium Development Goals and the aims of the Millennium Declaration, and for the vision set out above to become reality for all children.

The targets of the 1990 Innocenti Declaration and the 2002 Global Strategy for Infant and Young Child Feeding remain the foundation for action. While remarkable progress has been made, much more needs to be done.

We therefore issue this call for action so that:

All parties:
- Empower women in their own right, and as mothers and providers of breastfeeding support and information to other women.
- Support breastfeeding as the norm for feeding infants and young children.
- Highlight the risks of artificial feeding and the implications for health and development throughout the life course.
- Ensure the health and nutritional status of women throughout all stages of life.
- Protect breastfeeding in emergencies, including supporting uninterrupted breastfeeding and appropriate complementary feeding and avoiding general distribution of breastmilk substitutes.
- Implement the HIV and Infant Feeding: Framework for Priority Action, including protecting, promoting, and supporting breastfeeding for the general population while providing counseling and support for HIV-positive women.

All governments:

- Establish or strengthen national infant and young child feeding and breastfeeding authorities, coordinating committees, and oversight groups that are free from commercial influence and other conflicts of interest.
- Revitalize the Baby-Friendly Hospital Initiative (BFHI), maintaining the global criteria as the minimum requirement for all facilities, expanding the Initiative's application to include maternity, neonatal and child health services, and community-based support for lactating women and caregivers of young children.
- Implement all provisions of the International Code of Marketing of Breast-milk Substitutes and subsequent relevant World Health Assembly resolutions in their entirety as a minimum requirement, and establish sustainable enforcement mechanisms to prevent and/or address noncompliance.
- Adopt maternity protection legislation and other measures that facilitate 6 months of exclusive breastfeeding for women employed in all sectors, with urgent attention to the nonformal sector.
- Ensure that appropriate guidelines and skill acquisition regarding infant and young child feeding are included in both preservice and in-service training of all healthcare staff, to enable them to implement infant and young child feeding policies, and to provide a high standard of breastfeeding management and counseling to support mothers toward optimal breastfeeding and complementary feeding.
- Ensure that all mothers are aware of their rights and have access to support, information, and counseling in breastfeeding and complementary feeding from health workers and peer groups.
- Establish sustainable systems for monitoring infant and young child feeding patterns and trends, and use this information for advocacy and programming.

- Encourage the media to provide positive images of optimal infant and young child feeding, to support breastfeeding as the norm, and to participate in social activities such as World Breastfeeding Week.
- Take measures to protect populations, especially pregnant and breastfeeding mothers, from environmental contaminants and chemical residues.
- Identify and allocate sufficient resources to fully implement actions called for in the Global Strategy for Infant and Young Child Feeding.
- Monitor progress in appropriate infant and young child feeding practices and report periodically, including as provided in the Convention on the Rights of the Child.

All manufacturers and distributors of products within the scope of the international Code:
- Ensure full compliance with all provisions of the International Code and subsequent relevant World Health Assembly resolutions in all countries, independently of any other measures taken to implement the Code.
- Ensure that all processed foods for infants and young children meet applicable Codex Alimentarius standards.

Multilateral, bilateral, and international financial institutions:
- Recognize that optimal breastfeeding and complementary feeding are essential to achieving the long-term physical, intellectual, and emotional health of all populations, and therefore the attainment of the Millennium Development Goals and other development initiatives, and that inappropriate feeding practices and their consequences are major obstacles to poverty reduction and sustainable socioeconomic development.
- Identify and budget for sufficient financial resources and expertise to support governments in formulating, implementing, monitoring,

and evaluating their policies and programs on optimal infant and young child feeding, including the BFHI.

- Increase technical guidance and support for national capacity building in all target areas set forth in the Global Strategy for Infant and Young Child Feeding.
- Support operational research to fill information gaps and improve programming.
- Encourage the inclusion of programs to improve breastfeeding and complementary feeding in poverty-reduction strategies and health sector development plans.

Public interest nongovernmental organizations:

- Give greater priority to protecting, promoting, and supporting optimal feeding practices, including relevant training of health and community workers, and increase effectiveness through cooperation and mutual support.
- Draw attention to activities that are incompatible with the Code's principles and aims so that violations can be effectively addressed in accordance with national legislation, regulations, or with other suitable measures.

Reproduced with permission from World Health Organization, & UNICEF. (2005, November 22). Innocenti Declaration 2005 on Infant and Young Child Feeding. Retrieved from http://www.ers.usda.gov/publications /fanrr13/fanrr13.pdf.

APPENDICES

APPENDIX W

Glossary

A

AAP Acronym for the American Academy of Pediatrics.

ABM Acronym for the Academy of Breastfeeding Medicine; also acronym for "artificial baby milk" (infant formula).

abscess A localized collection of pus, associated with inflammatory (and sometimes infective) processes.

ACOG Acronym for the American Congress of Obstetricians and Gynecologists.

AGA Acronym for "appropriate for gestational age."

alternate massage A method of breast compression used during feeding to increase the flow of milk to the baby. The mother compresses the breast with her hand when the baby pauses in sucking.

alveoli Small glands in the breast that produce breastmilk.

amenorrhea The absence of menstrual cycle.

anemia A condition in which the blood is deficient in red blood cells, in hemoglobin, or in total volume.

anomaly An unusual condition or abnormality.

AOM Acronym for "acute otitis media" (middle ear infection).

Apgar A 10-point score determined for the newborn baby at birth, reflecting the health of the baby at that time. The name of the score is both the last name of the inventor, Dr. Virginia Apgar, and an acronym for the criteria scored: Appearance, Pulse, Grimace, Activity, and Respiration.

apnea Temporary cessation of breathing.

areola Darkened area around the nipple.

asymmetric breasts Breasts that are not similar in appearance. See also **discrepant breasts**.

asymmetric latch Optimal attachment to the breast, where the baby's lips are not centered in relationship to the areola, but rather vertically off-centered with the baby's chin and lower lip closer to the edge of the areola than the baby's upper lip.

at-breast supplementer Fine plastic tubing, with one end attached to a container holding expressed human milk or formula and the other end taped to the breast.

atopy An allergy for which there is a genetic predisposition, such as asthma, eczema, or rhinitis.

B

BF Acronym for "breastfed" or "breastfeeding."

BFHI The UNICEF Baby-Friendly Hospital Initiative, an international program recognizing hospitals and birth centers that implement the Ten Steps to Successful Breastfeeding.

bilirubin By-product of the breakdown of the hemoglobin portion of red blood cells.

bilirubin encephalopathy Damage to the brain and central nervous system related to hyperbilirubinemia (jaundice), also known as "kernicterus."

bleb A firm, small, white spot near the nipple pore opening containing accumulated milk solids. Also referred to as a milk blister.

block nursing A pattern of feeding used to deal with an overly abundant milk supply. In block feeding, the mother offers the baby only one breast for one, two, or three feedings to generate mild local pressure to slow down milk production. Then she offers the other breast for a block of time.

blocked milk duct A condition in which milk from one part of the breast does not flow well and forms a lump of thickened milk that blocks the milk duct.

brachial plexus injury Decreased movement or sensation in the arm caused by injury to the bundle of nerves passing through the shoulder area. This may be caused during birth by pressure to the shoulder area.

bradycardia Slow heart rate (less than 100 beats per minute in an infant).

breast abscess Area in the breast that feels hot and painful and is full of fluid. It results from unresolved mastitis.

breast compression A method used during feeding to increase the flow of milk to the baby. The mother gently squeezes her breast when the baby pauses in sucking. Also called "alternate massage."

breastmilk jaundice Jaundice occurring in the breastfed infant after 10–14 days of life. The cause of breastmilk jaundice is unknown and the incidence is less than 1 percent.

brucellosis Bacterial infection from contact with animals carrying *Brucella* bacteria. Infection causes an undulating fever that spikes in waves.

C

Candida A family of parasitic fungi occurring especially in the mouth, vagina, and intestinal tract. They are usually benign but can become pathogenic and include the causative agent (*Candida albicans*) of thrush.

caput succedaneum Swelling of the soft tissues of a newborn baby's scalp that develops as the baby travels through the birth canal.

CDC Acronym for the U.S. Department of Health and Human Services Centers for Disease Control and Prevention.

cephalohematoma A lump that rises on the head of a newborn within hours of birth due to bleeding beneath the bones of the skull.

chorioamniotis Inflammation of the fetal membranes due to infection.

circumoral cyanosis Blue coloration of the lips, usually due to inadequate circulation.

clavicle Collar bone, occasionally fractured during the birth process.

cleft lip A congenital birth defect causing division or split in the lip.

cleft palate A congenital birth defect causing a division or opening in the roof of the mouth.

CMV Acronym for "cytomegalovirus." See **cytomegalovirus**.

collaborative feeding Phase of breastfeeding following self-attached feeding, in which the mother and baby are learning to manage feeding together.

colostrum The first milk, produced in the breasts by the 7th month of pregnancy. Colostrum is thick, sticky, and clear to yellowish in color; is high in protein and vitamin A; and causes a laxative effect, thus helping the baby to pass meconium. Immunoglobulins (mostly IgA) in colostrum provide an anti-infective protection to the baby.

complementary feeding The feeding of both human milk and solid or semi-solid food to a child between 6 and 23 months of age.

contraindication A condition or factor that makes something inadvisable.

Cooper's ligaments The triangular-shaped ligaments underlying the breasts.

cradle hold Breastfeeding position in which the mother holds the baby on her lap with his or her head resting on the mother's forearm directly in front of the breast. Also called the Madonna hold.

craniofacial Involving the head and skull.

crib death The unexpected and sudden death of a seemingly normal and healthy infant that occurs during sleep and with no physical evidence of disease. The origin is unknown. Also called sudden infant death syndrome (SIDS).

cyanosis Blue coloration of the skin, usually due to inadequate circulation.

cytomegalovirus A virus of the herpes family that is relatively harmless in adults but can cause severe systemic infection in infants, particularly those born prematurely.

D

dehydration A condition in which the infant is not receiving adequate fluids or is unable to maintain adequate hydration for another metabolic reason. In addition to the symptoms of actual dehydration, vomiting, diarrhea, and nausea could be adding to or causing the dehydration. This problem can become grave for the young infant. Symptoms include:

- Dry or sticky mouth.
- Low or no urine output.
- Concentrated urine that appears dark yellow.
- Nonproduction of tears.
- Sunken eyes.
- Markedly sunken fontanelles in an infant.
- Lethargy or coma (with severe dehydration).

diabetes mellitus A group of diseases in which the body has difficulty managing stable blood sugar.

discordant twins Twin pairs with a marked difference in size at birth.

discrepant breasts A condition in which a woman's breasts are markedly different in size and/or shape. This is associated with potential milk supply problems. Also called "asymmetric" breasts.

Down syndrome A congenital condition characterized by moderate to severe mental retardation. Also called trisomy 21.

dyad A group of two. In lactation terms, usually refers to the nursing mother and baby.

Duarte galactosemia A variant of galactosemia with generally milder complications.

E

EBF Acronym for "exclusively breastfed" *or* "exclusive breastfeeding." See **exclusive breastfeeding**.

EBM Acronym for "expressed breastmilk."

EBMF Acronym for "exclusive breastmilk feeding." See **exclusive breastmilk feeding**.

eczema A noncontagious inflammation of the skin, characterized chiefly by redness, itching, and the outbreak of lesions that may become encrusted and scaly.

edema Swelling from excess accumulation of fluids in the cells or tissues of the body.

ELBW Acronym for "extremely low birth weight." See **extremely low birthweight infant**.

engorgement Swelling in the breast that blocks milk flow; caused by inadequate or infrequent milk removal. The breast will be hot and painful and will look tight and shiny. With severe engorgement, milk production may stop.

everted nipple A nipple that turns outward when stimulated.

exclusive breastfeeding (EBF) The feeding of mother's milk as an infant's only food source. The World Health Organization (2008) indicates babies included in this category may also be receiving oral rehydration solution, vitamins and minerals, and/or other oral medications, but may not receive any other foods or fluids.

exclusive breastmilk feeding (EBMF) A term used by The Joint Commission (2011) to describe those babies who are receiving only human milk.

extremely low birthweight infant (ELBW) An infant with a birth weight < 1,000 grams (2.2 pounds).

F

failure to thrive (FTT) A condition in which baby's growth is inadequate and requires medical evaluation.

feeding cues Infant behaviors that indicate an interest in eating, including rapid eye movement, movement of hands near the face, rooting and seeking motions, and other behaviors.

flat nipple A nipple that everts in response to stimulation but is otherwise not projected.

follicle A small cavity or sac.

fontanelles The openings between skull plates in the infant. These are also referred to as "soft spots."

foremilk The milk that is expressed from the breast at the beginning of a breastfeed.

frenulum Membrane that supports or restricts the movement of a body part. For example, the lingual frenulum supports the tongue; the labial frenulum supports the lips.

FTT Acronym for "failure to thrive." See **failure to thrive**.

G

G6PD Acronym for "Glucose 6-phosphate dehydrogenase deficiency." See **Glucose-6-phosphate dehydrogenase deficiency**.

galactocele A milk-filled cyst in the breast, most likely caused by an obstructed duct.

galactogogue Foods or drinks given to the mother that are believed to increase milk production.

galactose A simple sugar that is a portion of lactose; the sugar present in milk.

galactosemia Congenital metabolic disorder causing inability of the body to use the simple sugar galactose, causing accumulation of galactose 1-phosphate in the body, which results in damage to the liver, central nervous system, and other body systems with permanent, even fatal, outcomes.

gape A wide opening of the mouth (ideally 140°–160°).

gastrointestinal Having to do with the stomach and intestinal tract.

GDM Acronym for "gestational diabetes mellitus." See **gestational diabetes mellitus**.

gestational Regarding the period from conception to birth.

gestational diabetes mellitus (GDM) A form of diabetes that occurs in pregnancy.

glucose-6-phosphate dehydrogenase deficiency (G6PD) A hereditary metabolic enzyme deficiency that leads to mild destruction of red blood cells and jaundice when the individual is ill or exposed to substances ranging from fava beans to sulfa drugs and beyond.

GI Acronym for "gastrointestinal." See **gastrointestinal**.

Goldsmith's sign The association of a baby's persistent refusal of one breast with possible breast cancer in the mother.

H

hematoma A blood-filled swelling resulting from a broken blood vessel.

hindmilk The milk expressed from the breast toward the end of a feed.

HIV Acronym for "human immunodeficiency virus." See **Human Immunodeficiency Virus**.

HM Acronym for "human milk."

HMF Acronym for "human milk fortifier."

HTLV Acronym for "human T-cell lymphotropic virus."

Human Immunodeficiency Virus (HIV) A group of retroviruses, especially HIV-1, that infect and destroy helper T-cells of the immune system, causing the marked reduction in their numbers that is diagnostic of Acquired Immune Deficiency Syndrome (AIDS). Also called AIDS virus.

hyperbilirubinemia High levels of bilirubin in the blood. See also **jaundice**.

hyperthyroidism Increased activity of the thyroid gland, leading to excess production of thyroid hormone.

hypoglycemia Low blood sugar.

hypothyroidism Decreased activity of the thyroid gland, leading to decreased production of thyroid hormone.

hypothermia Low body temperature.

hypotonia Low muscle tone.

I

IDDM Acronym for insulin-dependent diabetes mellitus. Also called type 1 diabetes mellitus.

immunoglobulin Group of proteins that provide immunity, including:

- **IgA** Causes passive systemic immune protection, blocks the adhesion of microbial pathogens onto the intestinal wall, and forms antibodies against bacteria and viruses.
- **IgD** Forms antibodies against bacteria.
- **IgE** Combines with antigens in the gut lumen and releases chemical mediators that cause increased vascular permeability.
- **IgG** Can activate complements, and acts against bacteria and viruses.
- **IgM** Forms antibodies against bacteria and viruses; retains activity after traversing the intestinal canal.

induced lactation Process of establishing a milk supply in a woman who has not given birth.

inflammation A localized reaction of tissue to the presence of items perceived to be foreign or other irritation, injury, or infection characterized by pain, redness, and swelling.

inverted nipple A nipple that turns inward when stimulated.

IUGR Acronym for "intrauterine growth restriction."

J

jaundice Condition that results when red blood cells break down faster than the liver can handle, causing a yellow color of the skin. In the newborn, normal physiologic jaundice is caused by the immaturity of the liver.

K

kernicterus Damage to the brain and central nervous system related to hyperbilirubinemia (jaundice), also known as bilirubin encephalopathy.

L

lactiferous duct See **milk duct**.

lactogenesis Stages of development of the milk production process.

lactose A disaccharide (sugar) found only in mammalian milk.

late preterm infant (LPTI) An infant born between 34 0/7 and 36 6/7 weeks.

LBW Acronym for "low birth weight" (infant weighs less than 2,500 grams [5 pounds, 8 ounces]).

LCP Acronym for "lactation care provider."

letdown reflex The spontaneous ejection of milk from the breast. See also **milk ejection reflex**.

LGA Acronym for "large for gestational age."

low birth weight infant (LBW) Infant weighing less than 2,500 grams (< 5 pounds, 8 ounces) at birth.

LPTI Acronym for "late preterm infant." See **late preterm infant**.

M

malaise A sense of weakness or illness.

malnutrition A state in which the baby is either overfed, underfed, or unable to correctly utilize the food he or she is receiving.

mastitis Inflammation in the breast causing localized tenderness, redness, and heat. Mother may have a fever; feel tired, achy, or nauseous; or have a headache. Mastitis may or may not be an infective process.

meconium First stool of a newborn, varying from greenish black to light brown with a tarry consistency.

methicillin-resistant *Staphylococcus aureus* **(MRSA)** A bacterial infection that is very resistant to many antibiotics.

microcephaly Abnormal smallness of the head.

milk duct Narrow tube structure that carries milk to the nipple.

milk ejection reflex Reflex initiated by the production of the hormone oxytocin that causes the contraction of myoepithelial cells, ejecting milk from the breast.

mitigate To alleviate or make milder.

Montgomery glands Small tubercles in the areola of the breast that contain both sebaceous and mammary lobes. These glands become more marked in pregnancy and secrete a fluid that lubricates the nipple area.

Moro reflex A response present in the normal infant from the third trimester through the 4th or 5th month after birth. When pulled up from a lying position and then released, the infant will spread its arms, then fold them back to the body, usually crying.

MRSA Acronym for "methycillin-resistant *Staphylococcus-aureus*." See **methicillin-resistant** *Staphylococcus aureus*.

mucosa The lining of body cavities that produces mucus (a viscous secretion containing mucin).

multipara ("multip") A woman who has given birth to multiple babies.

myoepithelial cells Smooth muscle cells that encircle the alveoli and ducts of the breast. Contraction of these cells causes the outward flow of milk.

N

NCHS Acronym for the CDC's National Center for Health Statistics.

nine stages The nine instinctive behavioral stages newborn babies go through in the first hours after birth.

nonnutritive sucking Sucking that causes little or no milk secretion, associated with eight or more sucks per swallow.

normal fullness Breast fullness that occurs when the milk is "coming in." Extra blood and lymph are brought to the breast. The breasts may feel warm, full, and heavy.

NSAIDs Acronym for "non-steroidal anti-inflammatory drugs" (e.g., ibuprofen).

nutritive sucking Sucking that causes milk flow, typically thought of as one or two sucks per swallow.

O

otitis media Middle ear infection.

oversupply A condition of excess milk production.

oxytocin Hormone that contracts the cells around the alveoli and sends milk down the ducts and out the nipple pores, causing milk ejection (aka, "letdown").

P

patent Refers to structures such as to milk ducts that are connected or open, rather than closed.

PCOS Acronym for "polycystic ovarian syndrome." See **polycystic ovarian syndrome**.

perinatal Around the time of birth, both pre- and postpartum.

pH A measure of acidity/alkalinity of a substance expressed on a scale of 0 to 14, where 0 is the most acidic, 7 is neutral, and 14 is the most alkaline (basic).

phenylalanine An essential amino acid.

phenylketonuria (PKU) An inherited disease resulting in the inability to digest phenylalanine. People with this diagnosis must avoid phenylalanine due to the risk of brain damage.

Pierre Robin sequence A group of malformations of the face that are present from birth. Effects of this sequence can include small lower jaw, clefts of the palate, and problems with tongue coordination and breathing.

pituitary infarct Death of an area of tissue in the pituitary gland, which is found in the brain.

PKU Acronym for "phenylketonuria." See **phenylketonuria**.

polycystic ovarian syndrome (PCOS) A hormonal condition among women that is a major cause of infertility.

postpartum adjustment disorder (PPAD) Mood changes occurring to a woman in the first year after giving birth.

postpartum depression (PPD) Depression occurring in the first year postpartum.

PPAD Acronym for "postpartum adjustment disorder." See **postpartum adjustment disorder**.

PPD Acronym for "postpartum depression." See **postpartum depression**.

predominant breastfeeding The feeding of both mother's milk as well as water, water-based drinks, ritual foods (such as teas), oral rehydration solution, vitamins, minerals, and oral medications to the baby.

premature infant A baby born before 37 weeks' gestation.

preterm infant A baby born before 37 weeks' gestation.

primipara ("primip") A woman who is giving birth for the first time.

progesterone A hormone produced by the placenta during pregnancy.

progestin A synthetic form of progesterone, used in many birth control methods.

prolactin Hormone that stimulates the production of milk.

R

Raynaud's syndrome A medical condition associated with vasoconstriction and reduced blood flow to an extremity of the body in response to cold stress.

relactation Process of reestablishing adequate milk production in a mother who has a greatly reduced milk production or who has stopped breastfeeding.

reverse cycle nursing Description of a feeding pattern in which the mother and baby sleep in close proximity and nurse during the night; the mother then goes to work in the morning, and the baby sleeps most of the day.

rooming-in A bonding approach in which the mother and baby share the same hospital room, beginning as soon as possible after birth.

rooting reflex Natural instinct of the newborn to turn his or her head toward the nipple and open his or her mouth when the mouth area is gently stroked with the nipple.

S

secondhand smoke Tobacco smoke that is breathed from being in the presence of others who are smoking.

self-attached Referring to the baby's ability to find, attach to, and suckle from the breast during the first weeks postpartum.

sepsis Severe infection in the bloodstream.

SF Acronym for "soy formula" or "soy fed."

SGA Acronym for "small for gestational age."

Sheehan's syndrome Damage to the pituitary gland (caused by postpartum hemorrhage), resulting in the inability to produce pituitary hormones, including prolactin.

SIDS Acronym for "sudden infant death syndrome." See **crib death**.

skin to skin The practice of holding the infant so that his or her bare chest is against that of the mother or father (baby held under the parent's clothing and covered as needed for warmth). This technique has been demonstrated to help the baby regulate heart rate, respiratory rate, and body temperature, and facilitates early breastfeeding.

SNS Acronym for "supplemental nursing system," a type of at-breast supplementer.

stridor A high-pitched wheezing sound.

submucosal cleft An opening in the bone above the roof of the palate that is covered with normal skin lining and is therefore more difficult to identify.

sucking Drawing into the mouth by forming a partial vacuum with the lips and tongue.

supplementary feeding The giving of food other than breastmilk to an infant to replace breastmilk calories.

symptothermal A method of fertility awareness that relies on tracking calendar rhythm, basal body temperature, and other techniques such as cervical mucus.

T

tandem nursing Nursing two or more children not of the same pregnancy—for example, a newborn and a toddler.

Ten Steps to Successful Breastfeeding Guidelines developed by UNICEF and the World Health Organization that promote, protect, and support breastfeeding in facilities that provide maternity services and care for newborn infants. See also **BFHI**.

term infant A baby born at or after 37 weeks' gestation.

theca lutein cysts Benign growths in the ovaries.

thrush infection Infection caused by the yeast *Candida albicans* that the baby may contract through the birth canal. It may produce white patches and ulcers in the baby's mouth. The baby may then transmit the oral infection to the mother's breasts.

tongue tie Restriction of the tongue caused by a short or tight membrane of skin (frenulum) under the tongue.

torticollis Swelling of the muscles of the neck causing restricted ability to move the head.

U

UNICEF Acronym for the United Nations Children's Fund.

V

vasospasm Constriction of the blood vessels by tightening of the muscles around them, typically causing reduced blood flow through that area.

very low birthweight infant (VLBW) Weighing less than 1,500 grams (3.3 pounds).

VLBW Acronym for "very low birth weight." See **very low birthweight infant**.

W

whey A protein fraction of milk that is prominent in human milk.

WHO Acronym for the World Health Organization.

WIC Acronym for federal- and state-funded Special Supplemental Nutrition Program for Women, Infants & Children.

WNL Acronym for "within normal limits."

APPENDIX X

Conversions

1 milliliter (mL)	= 0.0338 fluid ounce (oz)
1 liter (L)	= 33.8148 ounces (oz)
1 gram (g)	= 0.03527 ounce (oz)
1 kilogram (kg)	= 2.2046 pounds (lbs)
38.4 degrees Centigrade	= 101 degrees Fahrenheit
1 fluid ounce (oz)	= 29.6 milliliters (mL)
1 quart (32 ounces)	= 907 milliliters (mL)
1 ounce (oz)	= 28.35 grams (g)
1 pound (lb)	= 0.45 kilograms (kg)

APPENDIX Y

Resources

HELPFUL ORGANIZATIONS

Academy of Breastfeeding Medicine (ABM)
Telephone: 1-914-740-2115
www.bfmed.org

Academy of Lactation Policy and Practice (ALPP)
Telephone: 1-508-833-1500
www.talpp.org

Academy of Nutrition and Dietetics
Telephone: 1-800-877-1600
www.eatright.org

American Academy of Family Physicians (AAFP)
Telephone: 1-913-906-6000
www.aafp.org

American Academy of Nursing
Telephone: 1-202-777-1170
www.aannet.org

American Academy of Pediatrics (AAP)
Telephone: 1-847-434-4000
www.aap.org

American Breastfeeding Institute
www.facebook.com/American-Breastfeeding-Institute-
176421862426503/timeline

278

American College of Nurse–Midwives (ACNM)
Telephone: 1-240-485-1800
www.midwife.org

American College of Osteopathic Pediatricians
Telephone: 1-804-565-6333
www.acopeds.org

American Congress of Obstetricians and Gynecologists
  (ACOG)
Telephone: 1-202-638-5577
www.acog.org

American Nurses Association
Telephone: 1-800-274-4262
nursingworld.org

American Public Health Association
Telephone: 1-202-777-2742
www.apha.org

Association of Maternal & Child Health Programs
Telephone: 1-202-775-0436
www.amchp.org

Association of State Public Health Nutritionists
Telephone: 1-814-255-2829
www.asphn.org

Association of Women's Health, Obstetric and Neonatal
  Nurses (AWHONN)
Telephone: 1-800-673-8499
www.awhonn.org

Baby Café USA
www.babycafeusa.org

Baby-Friendly USA, Inc. (BFUSA)
Telephone: 1-518-621-7982
www.babyfriendlyusa.org

Baby Milk Action
Telephone: +44 1223 464420 (United Kingdom)
www.babymilkaction.org

Best for Babes Foundation, Inc.
www.bestforbabes.org

Black Mothers' Breastfeeding Association
Telephone: 1-800-313-6141
www.bmbfa.org

BreastCancer.org
Telephone: 1-610-642-6550
www.breastcancer.org

Breastfeeding USA
www.breastfeedingusa.org

Carolina Global Breastfeeding Institute
Telephone: 1-919-966-0928
http://breastfeeding.sph.unc.edu

Centering Healthcare Institute
Telephone: 1-857-284-7570
www.centeringhealthcare.org

Coalition for Improving Maternity Services (CIMS)
Telephone: 1-866-424-3635
www.motherfriendly.org

Cochrane Collaboration
www.cochrane.org

Every Mother, Inc.
Telephone: 1-877-666-7226
www.everymother.org

FHI 360
Telephone: 1-919-544-7040
www.fhi360.org

Health Education Associates, Inc. (HEA)
Telephone: 1-508-888-8044
www.healthed.cc

HealthConnect One
Telephone: 1-312-243-4772
www.healthconnectone.org

Healthy Children Project (HCP)
Telephone: 1-508-888-8044
www.centerforbreastfeeding.org

Human Milk Banking Association of North America
(HMBANA)
Telephone: 1-817-810-9984
www.hmbana.org

International Baby Food Action Network (IBFAN)
Telephone: +41 22 7989164
www.ibfan.org

International Board of Lactation Consultant Examiners
(IBLCE)
Telephone: 1-703-560-7330
www.iblce.org

International Childbirth Education Association (ICEA)
Telephone: 1-919-863-9487
www.icea.org

International Lactation Consultant Association (ILCA)
Telephone: 1-919-861-5577
www.ilca.org

La Leche League International (LLLI)
Telephone: 1-312-646-6260
www.llli.org

Lactation Education Accreditation and Approval Review
    Committee (LEAARC)
Telephone: 1-919-459-6106
www.leaarc.org

Lactation Study Center, University of Rochester School of
    Medicine
Telephone: 1-585-275-0088, 8 am to 5 pm Eastern (health-
    care professionals only)
www.urmc.rochester.edu/childrens-hospital/neonatology
    /lactation.aspx

Lactnet (electronic discussion group for lactation
    professionals)
www.lsoft.com/scripts/wl.exe?SL1=LACTNET&H
    =COMMUNITY.LSOFT.com

Lamaze International
Telephone: 1-800-368-4404
www.lamaze.org

Medline Access
www.pubmed.gov

MomsRising
www.momsrising.org

National Alliance for Breastfeeding Advocacy (NABA)
www.naba-breastfeeding.org

National Association of Pediatric Nurse Practitioners
  (NAPNAP)
Telephone: 1-917-746-8300
www.napnap.org

National Black Nurses Association (NBNA)
Telephone: 1-301-589-3200
www.nbna.org

National Commission on Donor Milk Banking, American
  Breastfeeding Institute
Telephone: 1-508-888-9366

National Perinatal Association (NPA)
Telephone: 1-888-971-3295
www.nationalperinatal.org

National WIC Association (NWA)
Telephone: 1-202-232-5492
www.nwica.org

Public Citizen
Telephone: 1-202-588-1000
www.citizen.org

Reaching Our Sisters Everywhere (ROSE)
Telephone: 1-404-719-4297
www.breastfeedingrose.org

United Nations Children's Fund (UNICEF)
Telephone: 1-212-326-7000
www.unicef.org

United States Breastfeeding Committee (USBC)
Telephone: 1-773-359-1549
www.usbreastfeeding.org

United States Lactation Consultant Association (USLCA)
Telephone: 1-919-861-4543
www.uslca.org

U.S. Department of Agriculture (USDA)
Food and Nutrition Service WIC
Telephone: 1-703-305-2062
www.fns.usda.gov

U.S. Department of Health and Human Services
(USDHHS)
Centers for Disease Control and Prevention (CDC)
Telephone: 1-800-232-4636
www.cdc.gov/breastfeeding

U.S. Department of Health and Human Services
Maternal Child Health Bureau (MCHB)
Telephone: 1-800-221-9393
www.mchb.hrsa.gov

U.S. Department of Health and Human Services
Office of Women's Health (OWH)
Telephone: 1-202-690-7650
www.womenshealth.gov

U.S. Food and Drug Administration (FDA)
Telephone: 1-888-INFO-FDA
www.fda.gov
To report equipment damage, search the FDA
Manufacturer and User Facility Device Experience
(MAUDE) Database

Wellstart International
www.wellstart.org

Women-Inspired Systems' Enrichment
Telephone: 1-919-630-4460
www.wiseqi.org

World Alliance for Breastfeeding Advocacy (WABA)
www.waba.org.my

World Health Organization (WHO)
www.who.org

AT-BREAST FEEDING RESOURCES
Lact-Aid Nursing Trainer System
www.lact-aid.com

Medela Supplemental Nurser System
www.medela.com

MEDICATION SAFETY RESOURCES
Infant Risk Center
Telephone: 1-806-352-2519
www.infantrisk.com

Lactation Study Center, University of Rochester School of Medicine

Telephone: 1-585-275-0088, 8 am to 5 pm Eastern (health-care professionals only)

LactMed (U.S. National Library of Medicine searchable database on drugs in lactation)

https://toxnet.nlm.nih.gov/newtoxnet/lactmed.htm

APPENDIX Z

Pediatric Warning Signs

Seek emergent medical care if any of these signs is present:

- Exclusively breastfed newborn baby with less than one stool per day.
- Meconium bowel movements after day 5 of life.
- No urine in 6 hours.
- No interest in feeding for more than 6 hours.
- Dark-colored urine.
- Brick dust urine (uric acid crystals).
- Noticeably sunken fontanelles (soft spot on top of the head).
- Decreased activity.
- Severe lethargy (sleepiness) or irritability.
- Poor feeding.
- Fever.
- Sudden change in muscle tone (extremely floppy or stiff).
- Sudden disinterest in feeding.
- Unable to wake baby.
- Doesn't calm, even with cuddles.
- Circumoral cyanosis (blue-tinged skin around the mouth when crying or breathing).
- Advancing jaundice.

References

AAP Committee on Fetus & Newborn, & Adamkin, D. H. (2011). Postnatal glucose homeostasis in late-preterm and term infants. *Pediatrics, 127*(3), 575–579. http://doi.org/10.1542/peds.2010-3851

AAP Section on Breastfeeding. (2012). Breastfeeding and the use of human milk (2012). *Pediatrics, 129*(3), e827–e841. http://doi.org/10.1542/peds.2011-3552

Ahluwalia, I. B., Morrow, B., & Hsia, J. (2005). Why do women stop breastfeeding? Findings from the Pregnancy Risk Assessment and Monitoring System. *Pediatrics, 116*(6), 1408–1412. http://doi.org/10.1542/peds.2005-0013

Aljazaf, K., Hale, T. W., Ilett, K. F., Hartmann, P. E., Mitoulas, L. R., Kristensen, J. H., Hackett, L. P. (2003). Pseudoephedrine: Effects on milk production in women and estimation of infant exposure via breastmilk. *British Journal of Clinical Pharmacology, 56*(1), 18–24.

American Academy of Pediatrics (AAP). (2015, November 21). Amount and schedule of formula feedings. Retrieved January 23, 2016, from https://www.healthychildren.org/English/ages-stages/baby/feeding-nutrition/Pages/Amount-and-Schedule-of-Formula-Feedings.aspx

American Academy of Pediatrics, Subcommittee on Hyperbilirubinemia. (2004). Management of hyperbilirubinemia in the newborn infant 35 or more weeks of gestation. *Pediatrics, 114*(1), 297–316.

American Academy of Pediatrics, Task Force on Sudden Infant Death Syndrome. (2005). The changing concept of sudden infant death syndrome: Diagnostic coding shifts, controversies regarding the sleeping environment, and new variables to consider in reducing risk. *Pediatrics, 116*(5), 1245–1255. http://doi.org/10.1542/peds.2005-1499

Amir, L. H. (2007). Medicines and breastfeeding: Information is available on safe use. *The Medical Journal of Australia, 186*(9), 485.

Amir, L. H., Forster, D. A., Lumley, J., & McLachlan, H. (2007). A descriptive study of mastitis in Australian breastfeeding women: Incidence and determinants. *BioMed Central Public Health, 7*, 62. http://doi.org/10.1186/1471-2458-7-62

Andersen, A. N., Lund-Andersen, C., Larsen, J. F., Christensen, N. J., Legros, J. J., Louis, F., . . . Molin, J. (1982). Suppressed prolactin but normal neurophysin levels in cigarette smoking breast-feeding women. *Clinical Endocrinology, 17*(4), 363–368.

Anderson, J. E., Held, N., & Wright, K. (2004). Raynaud's phenomenon of the nipple: A treatable cause of painful breastfeeding. *Pediatrics, 113*(4), e360–e364.

Aono, T., Shioji, T., Shoda, T., & Kurachi, K. (1977). The initiation of human lactation and prolactin response to suckling. *The Journal of Clinical Endocrinology and Metabolism, 44*(6), 1101–1106.

Baby-Friendly USA. (n.d.). The Ten Steps to Successful Breastfeeding. Retrieved March 25, 2016, from http://www.babyfriendlyusa.org/about-us/baby-friendly-hospital-initiative/the-ten-steps

Baby-Friendly USA, Inc. (2010, June 10). Guidelines and evaluation criteria for facilities seeking Baby-Friendly designation. Retrieved from https://www.babyfriendlyusa.org/get-started/the-guidelines-evaluation-criteria

Batstra, L., Neeleman, J., & Hadders-Algra, M. (2003). Can breast feeding modify the adverse effects of smoking during pregnancy on the child's cognitive development? *Journal of Epidemiology and Community Health, 57*(6), 403–404.

Beauchamp, G. K., & Mennella, J. A. (2011). Flavor perception in human infants: Development and functional significance. *Digestion, 83*(Suppl. 1), 1–6. http://doi.org/10.1159/000323397

Blair, P., & Inch, S. (2011). The health professional's guide to: "Caring for your baby at night." UNICEF UK. Retrieved from http://www.unicef.org.uk/documents/baby_friendly/leaflets/hps_guide_to_coping_at_night_final.pdf

Branch-Elliman, W., Golen, T. H., Gold, H. S., Yassa, D. S., Baldini, L. M., & Wright, S. B. (2012). Risk factors for *Staphylococcus aureus* postpartum breast abscess. *Clinical Infectious Diseases, 54*(1), 71–77. http://doi.org/10.1093/cid/cir751

Brown, K., Dewey, K., & Allen, L. (1998). *Complementary feeding of young children in developing countries: A review of current scientific knowledge*. World Health Organization. Retrieved from http://www.popline.org/node/532060

Cadwell, K., & Turner-Maffei, C. (2004). *Case studies in breastfeeding: Problem-solving skills & strategies*. Sudbury, MA: Jones and Bartlett Publishers.

Cadwell, K., Turner-Maffei, C., Blair, A., Brimdyr, K., & McInerney, Z. M. (2004). Pain reduction and treatment of sore nipples in nursing mothers. *The Journal of Perinatal Education, 13*(1), 29–35. http://doi.org/10.1624/105812404X109375

Carfoot, S., Williamson, P., & Dickson, R. (2005). A randomised controlled trial in the north of England examining the effects of skin-to-skin care on breast feeding. *Midwifery, 21*(1), 71–79. http://doi.org/10.1016/j.midw.2004.09.002

Centers for Disease Control and Prevention. (2009a, October 20). Breastfeeding: Hepatitis B and C infections. Retrieved April 20, 2015, from http://www.cdc.gov/breastfeeding/disease /hepatitis.htm

Centers for Disease Control and Prevention. (2009b, October 20). Breastfeeding: What to do if an infant or child is mistakenly fed another woman's expressed breast milk. Retrieved January 23, 2016, from http://www.cdc.gov/breastfeeding /recommendations/other_mothers_milk.htm

Centers for Disease Control & Prevention. (2010). Breastfeeding: Proper handling and storage of human milk. Retrieved January 25, 2016, from http://www.cdc.gov/breastfeeding /recommendations/handling_breastmilk.htm

Centers for Disease Control and Prevention. (2011a). Update to CDC's U.S. Medical Eligibility Criteria for Contraceptive Use, 2010: Revised recommendations for the use of contraceptive methods during the postpartum period. *MMWR. Morbidity and Mortality Weekly Report, 60*(26), 878–883.

Centers for Disease Control and Prevention. (2011b, June 30). Breastfeeding: Healthy People 2020 objectives for the nation. Retrieved January 23, 2016, from http://www.cdc.gov /breastfeeding/policy/hp2010.htm?topicId=26

Centers for Disease Control & Prevention. (2015). Breastfeeding: Diseases and conditions. Retrieved January 22, 2016, from http://www.cdc.gov/breastfeeding/disease/index.htm

Christensen, A. F., Al-Suliman, N., Nielsen, K. R., Vejborg, I., Severinsen, N., Christensen, H., Nielsen, M. B. (2005). Ultrasound-guided drainage of breast abscesses: Results in 151 patients. *British Journal of Radiology, 78*(927), 186–188.

Christensson, K., Siles, C., Moreno, L., Belaustequi, A., De La Fuente, P., Lagercrantz, H., . . . Winberg, J. (1992). Temperature, metabolic adaptation and crying in healthy full-term newborns cared for skin-to-skin or in a cot. *Acta Paediatrica, 81*(6-7), 488–493.

Cooper, W. O., Atherton, H. D., Kahana, M., & Kotagal, U. R. (1995). Increased incidence of severe breastfeeding malnutrition and hypernatremia in a metropolitan area. *Pediatrics, 96*(5 Pt 1), 957–960.

Cox, J. L., Holden, J. M., & Sagovsky, R. (1987). Detection of postnatal depression. Development of the 10-item Edinburgh Postnatal Depression Scale. *British Journal of Psychiatry, 150,* 782–786.

Dewey, K. (2003). Guiding principles for complementary feeding of the breastfed child. Pan American Health Organization. Retrieved from http://www.who.int/nutrition/publications /guiding_principles_compfeeding_breastfed.pdf

Dodd, R. (2005). *Health and the millennium development goals: 2000, 2005 keep the promise, 2015*. Geneva, Switzerland: World Health Organization.

Feher, S. D., Berger, L. R., Johnson, J. D., & Wilde, J. B. (1989). Increasing breast milk production for premature infants with a relaxation/imagery audiotape. *Pediatrics, 83*(1), 57–60.

Fein, S. B., Mandal, B., & Roe, B. E. (2008). Success of strategies for combining employment and breastfeeding. *Pediatrics, 122*(Suppl. 2), S56–S62. http://doi.org/10.1542/peds.2008-1315g

Fetherston, C. (1998). Risk factors for lactation mastitis. *Journal of Human Lactation, 14*(2), 101–109.

Flaherman, V. J., Gay, B., Scott, C., Avins, A., Lee, K. A., & Newman, T. B. (2012). Randomised trial comparing hand expression with breast pumping for mothers of term newborns feeding poorly. *Archives of Disease in Childhood. Fetal and Neonatal Edition, 97*(1), F18–F23. http://doi.org/10.1136/adc.2010.209213

Food & Drug Administration, U. S. (2013). Buying and renting a breast pump. Retrieved January 22, 2016, from http://www.fda.gov/MedicalDevices/ProductsandMedicalProcedures/HomeHealthandConsumer/ConsumerProducts/BreastPumps/ucm061952.htm

Francis-Morrill, J., Heinig, M. J., Pappagianis, D., & Dewey, K. G. (2004). Diagnostic value of signs and symptoms of mammary candidosis among lactating women. *Journal of Human Lactation, 20*(3), 288–295; quiz 296–299. http://doi.org/10.1177/0890334404267226

Groër, M. W. (2005). Differences between exclusive breastfeeders, formula-feeders, and controls: A study of stress, mood, and endocrine variables. *Biological Research for Nursing, 7*(2), 106–117. http://doi.org/10.1177/1099800405280936

Hale, T. (2014). *Medications and mothers' milk 2014*. (16th ed.). Amarillo TX: Hale Pub L P.

Hale, T. W., Bateman, T. L., Finkelman, M. A., & Berens, P. D. (2009). The absence of *Candida albicans* in milk samples of women with clinical symptoms of ductal candidiasis. *Breastfeeding Medicine, 4*(2), 57–61. http://doi.org/10.1089/bfm.2008.0144

Han, S., & Hong, Y. G. (1999). The inverted nipple: Its grading and surgical correction. *Plastic and Reconstructive Surgery, 104*(2), 389–395; discussion 396–397.

Henderson, J. J., Hartmann, P. E., Newnham, J. P., & Simmer, K. (2008). Effect of preterm birth and antenatal corticosteroid treatment on lactogenesis II in women. *Pediatrics, 121*(1), e92–100. http://doi.org/10.1542/peds.2007-1107

Horta, B. L., Kramer, M. S., & Platt, R. W. (2001). Maternal smoking and the risk of early weaning: A meta-analysis. *American Journal of Public Health*, *91*(2), 304–307.

Hurst, N. M. (1996). Lactation after augmentation mammoplasty. *Obstetrics and Gynecology*, *87*(1), 30–34.

Institute of Medicine, Committee on Nutritional Status During Pregnancy and Lactation, Institute of Medicine. (1991). *Nutrition during lactation*. Washington, D.C.: National Academies Press.

Ip, S., Chung, M., Raman, G., Chew, P., Magula, N., DeVine, D., . . . Lau, J. (2007). Breastfeeding and maternal and infant health outcomes in developed countries. *Evidence Report/Technology Assessment*, (153), 1–186.

Ishii, H. (2009). Does breastfeeding induce spontaneous abortion? *The Journal of Obstetrics and Gynaecology Research*, *35*(5), 864–868. http://doi.org/10.1111/j.1447-0756.2009.01072.x

Jakobsson, I., & Lindberg, T. (1983). Cow's milk proteins cause infantile colic in breast-fed infants: A double-blind crossover study. *Pediatrics*, *71*(2), 268–271.

Kelmanson, I. A., Erman, L. V., & Litvina, S. V. (2002). Maternal smoking during pregnancy and behavioural characteristics in 2–4-month-old infants. *Klinische Pädiatrie*, *214*(6), 359–364. http://doi.org/10.1055/s-2002-35369

Kennedy, K. I. (2002). Efficacy and effectiveness of LAM. *Advances in Experimental Medicine and Biology*, *503*, 207–216.

Kramer, M. S., & Kakuma, R. (2004). Optimal duration of exclusive breastfeeding. *The Cochrane Database of Systematic Reviews*, *8*, CD003517. http://doi.org/10.1002/14651858.CD003517.pub2

Labbok, M., Cooney, K. A., & Coly, S. (1994). Guidelines: Breastfeeding, family planning, and the Lactational Amenorrhea Method–LAM. Washington, D.C.: Institute for Reproductive Health.

Li, R., Fein, S. B., Chen, J., & Grummer-Strawn, L. M. (2008). Why mothers stop breastfeeding: Mothers' self-reported reasons for stopping during the first year. *Pediatrics*, *122*(Suppl. 2), S69–76. http://doi.org/10.1542/peds.2008-1315i

Lucarelli, S., Di Nardo, G., Lastrucci, G., D'Alfonso, Y., Marcheggiano, A., Federici, T., . . . Cucciara, S. (2011). Allergic proctocolitis refractory to maternal hypoallergenic diet in exclusively breast-fed infants: A clinical observation. *BioMed Central Gastroenterology*, *11*, 82. http://doi.org/10.1186/1471-230X-11-82

Mangesi, L., & Dowswell, T. (2010). Treatments for breast engorgement during lactation. *The Cochrane Database of Systematic Reviews*, (9), CD006946. http://doi.org/10.1002/14651858.CD006946.pub2

Mennella, J. A., Jagnow, C. P., & Beauchamp, G. K. (2001). Prenatal and postnatal flavor learning by human infants. *Pediatrics, 107*(6), E88.

Montalto, M., & Lui, B. (2009). MRSA as a cause of postpartum breast abscess in infant and mother. *Journal of Human Lactation, 25*(4), 448–450. http://doi.org/10.1177/0890334409340777

Morton, J., Hall, J. Y., Wong, R. J., Thairu, L., Benitz, W. E., & Rhine, W. D. (2009). Combining hand techniques with electric pumping increases milk production in mothers of preterm infants. *Journal of Perinatology, 29*(11), 757–764. http://doi.org/10.1038/jp.2009.87

Morton, J., Wong, R. J., Hall, J. Y., Pang, W. W., Lai, C. T., Lui, J., . . . Rhine, W. D. (2012). Combining hand techniques with electric pumping increases the caloric content of milk in mothers of preterm infants. *Journal of Perinatology, 32*(10), 791–796. http://doi.org/10.1038/jp.2011.195

Nyqvist, K. H., Sjödén, P. O., & Ewald, U. (1999). The development of preterm infants' breastfeeding behavior. *Early Human Development, 55*(3), 247–264.

Ortiz, J., McGilligan, K., & Kelly, P. (2004). Duration of breast milk expression among working mothers enrolled in an employer-sponsored lactation program. *Pediatric Nursing, 30*(2), 111–119.

Phalen, A. (2011). Human Milk Intake in Preterm Infants: Correlation of the Preterm Infant Breastfeeding Behavior Scale (PIBBS) and Test Weighing. *School of Nursing Faculty Papers & Presentations*. Retrieved from http://jdc.jefferson.edu/nursfp/41

Pumberger, W., Pomberger, G., & Geissler, W. (2001). Proctocolitis in breast fed infants: A contribution to differential diagnosis of haematochezia in early childhood. *Postgraduate Medical Journal, 77*(906), 252–254.

Sachs, H. C., & Committee on Drugs. (2013). The transfer of drugs and therapeutics into human breast milk: An update on selected topics. *Pediatrics, 132*(3), e796–809. http://doi.org/10.1542/peds.2013-1985

Slusser, W. M., Lange, L., Dickson, V., Hawkes, C., & Cohen, R. (2004). Breast milk expression in the workplace: A look at frequency and time. *Journal of Human Lactation, 20*(2), 164–169. http://doi.org/10.1177/0890334404263731

Souto, G. C., Giugliani, E. R. J., Giugliani, C., & Schneider, M. A. (2003). The impact of breast reduction surgery on breastfeeding performance. *Journal of Human Lactation, 19*(1), 43–49; quiz 66–69, 120.

Stafford, I., Hernandez, J., Laibl, V., Sheffield, J., Roberts, S., & Wendel, G., Jr. (2008). Community-acquired methicillin-resistant

Staphylococcus aureus among patients with puerperal mastitis requiring hospitalization. *Obstetrics and Gynecology, 112*(3), 533–537. http://doi.org/10.1097/AOG.0b013e31818187b0

Taveras, E. M., Capra, A. M., Braveman, P. A., Jensvold, N. G., Escobar, G. J., & Lieu, T. A. (2003). Clinician support and psychosocial risk factors associated with breastfeeding discontinuation. *Pediatrics, 112*(1 Pt 1), 108–115.

The Joint Commission. (2015). Specifications manual for Joint Commission national quality measures (v2015B2). Retrieved January 23, 2016, from https://manual.jointcommission.org /releases/TJC2015B2/MIF0170.html

Thomassen, P., Johansson, V. A., Wassberg, C., & Petrini, B. (1998). Breast-feeding, pain and infection. *Gynecologic and Obstetric Investigation, 46*(2), 73–74.

Turner-Maffei, C., & Cadwell, K. (2015). Weight gain in young infants: Are our criteria for daily weight gain accurate? *Maternal & Child Nutrition, 11*(Suppl. 2), 119.

UNICEF. (2007). UNICEF in action: The International Code. Retrieved January 23, 2016, from http://www.unicef.org /programme/breastfeeding/code.htm

UNICEF Division of Communications. (2009). *Tracking progress on child and maternal nutrition.* New York, NY: Author.

UNICEF UK Baby-Friendly Initiative. (2011). Caring for your baby at night: A guide for parents. Retrieved from http:// www.unicef.org.uk/Documents/Baby_Friendly/Leaflets /caringatnight_web.pdf

U.S. Department of Health & Human Services. (2010). *Healthy People 2020* (No. ODPHP Publication No. B0132). Retrieved from http://www.healthypeople.gov/2020/TopicsObjectives2020 /pdfs/HP2020_brochure_with_LHI_508.pdf

U.S. Department of Health and Human Services. (2011). Healthy People 2020 Topics and Objectives: Maternal, Infant, and Child Health, MICH 20-24. U.S. Department of Health and Human Services, Office of the Surgeon General. Retrieved from http://www.healthypeople.gov/2020/topicsobjectives2020 /objectiveslist.aspx?topicid=26

U.S. Department of Health & Human Services. (2010). *Healthy People 2020* (No. ODPHP Publication No. B0132). Retrieved from http://www.healthypeople.gov/2020/TopicsObjectives2020 /pdfs/HP2020_brochure_with_LHI_508.pdf

Wessel, M. A., Cobb, J. C., Jackson, E. B., Harris, G. S., & Detwiler, A. C. (1954). Paroxysmal fussing in infancy, sometimes called colic. *Pediatrics, 14*(5), 421–435.

WHO, & UNICEF. (n.d.). Nutrition: Global strategy for infant and young child feeding. Retrieved June 14, 2014, from http://www.who.int/nutrition/topics/global_strategy_iycf/en

Widström, A.-M., Lilja, G., Aaltomaa-Michalias, P., Dahllöf, A., Lintula, M., & Nissen, E. (2011). Newborn behaviour to locate the breast when skin-to-skin: A possible method for enabling early self-regulation. *Acta Paediatrica, 100*(1), 79–85. http://doi.org/10.1111/j.1651-2227.2010.01983.x

Widström, A. M., & Thingström-Paulsson, J. (1993). The position of the tongue during rooting reflexes elicited in newborn infants before the first suckle. *Acta Paediatrica, 82*(3), 281–283.

World Health Organization. (1981). International Code of Marketing of Breast-milk Substitutes. World Health Organization. Retrieved from http://whqlibdoc.who.int/publications/9241541601.pdf

World Health Organization (2003). Global strategy for infant and young child feeding. Retrieved from http://whqlibdoc.who.int/publications/2003/9241562218.pdf

World Health Organization. (2008). *Indicators for Assessing Infant and Young Child Feeding. Part 1: Definitions.* Geneva, Switzerland: Author.

World Health Organization. (2009). *Acceptable medical reasons for use of breast-milk substitutes.* (No. WHO/NMH/NHD/09.01). Geneva, Switzerland: Author.

World Health Organization, & UNICEF. (1990, August 1). Innocenti Declaration on the Protection, Promotion and Support of Breastfeeding. UNICEF. Retrieved from http://www.unicef.org/programme/breastfeeding/innocenti.htm

World Health Organization, & UNICEF. (2005, November 22). Innocenti Declaration 2005 on Infant and Young Child Feeding. Retrieved from http://www.ers.usda.gov/publications/fanrr13/fanrr13.pdf

World Health Organization, & UNICEF. (2009). *Baby-Friendly Hospital Initiative: Revised, updated and expanded for integrated care. Section 1, Background and implementation.* Geneva, Switzerland: World Health Organization. Retrieved from http://whqlibdoc.who.int/publications/2009/9789241594967_eng.pdf

World Health Organization, UNICEF, & IBFAN. (2016). Marketing of breast-milk substitutes: National implementation of the international code. Status report 2016. Retrieved from http://www.who.int/nutrition/publications/infantfeeding/code_report2016/en

INDEX

Note: Figures are indicated by "f" following the page number.

A

AAP. *See* American Academy of Pediatrics
abscess, 71, 73–75, 172
active sleep state, 13
administrative staff, responsibilities of, 37–38
alcohol consumption, 87, 94
alternate massage/breast compression, 56, 96, 96f, 195–196, 195f
American Academy of Pediatrics (AAP), 81, 88, 140, 164, 199, 242
amniotic fluid, 86
analgesia, feeding issues from, 15, 120
anemia, 73
antenatal staff, responsibilities of, 30, 39
anti-inflammatory drugs, for breast and nipple issues, 10
antibiotics
  for breast and nipple issues, 10, 72–74
  breastfeeding affected by, 63
antiretroviral medication, 241
apnea, 142
artificial nipple, and bottle, 35–36, 98, 104, 156
aspiration pneumonia, 155
asymmetric breast, 85
asymmetric latch, 23, 24f, 48, 50
at-breast feeders, 3, 234, 285
augmentation, breast, 43–44, 126
Australian posture, 59, 59f, 89, 193, 194f, 224, 224f

B

baby. *See also* infants
Baby-Friendly facility designation, 28
Baby-Friendly Hospital Initiative (BFHI), 27–28, 251
Baby-Friendly USA, Inc., 28
baby-led weaning, 171
baby training plans, 93
baby weight loss table
  in grams, 214–216
  in lb-oz, 209–213
bacterial infection, of breast, 63–64
bed sharing, with baby, 94
BFHI. *See* Baby-Friendly Hospital Initiative
birth centers. *See* hospitals and birth centers
birth control, 174–177
birth defects, 143–153
birth injury, and feeding issues, 153–156
bleb, 64–66
block feeding, 89
blocked duct, 64–66
blood, in breastmilk, 55
blood level, of infant, 2
blue lips, during feeding, 110, 147–148
body language
  of baby, 109, 111, 188
  of mother, 188
bottle/cup refusal, 129–131
bottles, and artificial nipples, 35–36, 98, 104, 156
bowel movements, of baby, 58, 88, 217, 224
brachial plexus injury, 101, 113, 154
bradycardia, 142
bras, feeding and, 43, 51, 59, 63, 65, 72
breast and nipple issues, 43–75. *See also* engorgement; mastitis
  abscess, 71, 73–75, 172
  anti-inflammatory drugs for, 10
  antibiotics for, 10, 72–74
  bleb or milk blister, 64–66
  breast, storage capacity of, 77
  breast surgery. *See* breast surgery

breast and nipple issues
(*continued*)
nipple
artificial, 35–36, 98, 104, 156
everted, 46, 47*f*
flat, 46–48, 47*f*
infection of, 62
inverted, 40, 49–52, 49*f*,
218–219
shape, after latch-off, 14, 48,
51, 57, 223
shields, 48, 51, 57, 72
oversupply, 57–60, 88, 101,
223–225
pain
while actively feeding, 14,
52–57, 223
after breastfeeding, 60–62
relieving through expression
of breastmilk, 48, 60, 68
relieving through position
change, 52, 56, 58–59, 59*f*,
65, 224
plugged duct or caked breast,
59, 66, 69–71, 75
soreness, 169
yeast or thrush, 61–64
breast cancer, 10, 73, 75
breast compression
alternate massage, 56, 96, 96*f*,
195–196, 195*f*
to tamp supply, 59, 89
breast improvements. *See* breast
surgery
breast injury, 85, 218
breast pumps, 83–84, 91–92,
221, 231–233
flange of, 83–84
sharing, 233
breast shell, 51, 72
breast support, during nursing,
16–17, 17–18*f*
breast surgery, 40, 85, 125, 128,
218–219
augmentation, 43–44
reduction, 44–45
breast tissue, inadequate,
218–219
breast water baths, 67, 68*f*
breastfeeding, 150
ability to, 161–179
birth control compatibility
and, 174–177

during illness, 166–168
medication and, 163–166
multiple babies and, 177–179
during pregnancy, 169–171
smoking and, 161–163
weaning and, 171–174
artificial teat or pacifier, use
of, 35–36
benefits of, 1, 147, 158–159
cessation, early, 5
collaborative, 13–14, 16, 20
community support for, 39–41
contraindications to, 2, 150,
163, 165–166
defined, 4
on demand, encouraging, 35–36
discouraging factors for, 40
duration of, 1, 44
early days of, 14, 31, 66
eight-level, counseling process,
181–185, 182*f*
employer support for, 91–92
expectations of successful, 26
factors affecting duration of, 40
getting started at, 31–32
health implications of, 1, 30,
147, 158–159
history of, 5
informing women of benefits
of, 30
initiating after birth, 13–14,
31–32
instinctive nature of, 5
International Code of
Marketing of Breast-Milk
Substitutes compliance, 37
issues. *See* feeding issues
learning, 5, 13–14
management issues and, 77–94
feeding cues, 78–80, 78–80*f*
frequency of feeding, 77–78
insufficient milk supply, 82–85
mother's diet, 86–87
sleeping close to mother, 93–94
sleeping through night, 92–93
weight gain/loss of baby,
80–81, 87–90. *See also*
infants, weight
working and, 90–92
management strategies for, 39
newborns, food for, 33
normal. *See* normal
breastfeeding

observation checklist, 104, 107, 110, 112, 186–189
positions for, 190–194
  breast and nipple issues, alleviating, 52, 56–58, 59*f*, 64, 225
  feeding problems and, 100–101, 101*f*, 104, 113, 154–155
  management issues and, 89
  twins, triplets and multiples, 177–179
predominant, 3–4
in public, 174
public health aspects of, 1
refusing to, 95–106
rooming-in, practice of, 34
self-attached, 13
stopping early, 5
support for, 278–286
support groups, establishing, 36–37
teaching, 32–33
training for policy implementation, 29–30
written policy for, 28–29
breastmilk
bank, 3, 59, 81, 89
blood in, 55
daily volume requirement
  in grams and milliliters, 206–208
  in ounces, 201–205
diet affecting, 86–87
digestibility of, 77
diminishing supply, 82
discarding during work day, 91
expression of, 48
  instructions for, 230–233
  milk supply, increasing through, 83
  small quantity, 126–129
  working and, 90–91
factors to decrease, 159
flavor of, 86
freezing, 64, 239–240, 239*f*
handling of, 237–240, 239*f*
increasing of flow, 96, 218–222
insufficiency. *See* milk insufficiency
microwaving, 240
pumping, 83–84, 91–92, 221, 231–233
rate of, 108

refrigerating, 239–240, 239*f*
storing, 237–240, 239*f*
substitutes, 249–250. *See also* formula
supply adequacy. *See* milk supply adequacy
thawing, 239*f*, 240
transfer, 35, 40, 101–102, 197–198, 226–229
warming, 240
breathing, matching to mother's, 94
brucellosis, 167, 242
"Business Case for Breastfeeding" (Health Resources and Services Administration Office on Women's Health), 92

C

caffeine consumption, 87
caked breast, 66, 69–71, 75
caloric intake, of mother, 86
calorically deprived baby, 4, 51, 77, 82–83, 95
cancer
  breast, 10, 73, 75
  chemotherapy agents, 241
  skin, 3
Candida albicans, 62–64
caput succedaneum, 153
cardiac birth defect, and feeding issues, 108, 143–144
catch-up requirements
  in grams and milliliters, 206–208
  in ounces, 201–205
CDC. *See* Centers for Disease Control and Prevention
Center for Breastfeeding, 7, 199, 218, 221
Centers for Disease Control and Prevention (CDC), 88, 167, 241
cephalhematoma, 153–154
cesarean birth, 31, 66
checklist, feeding observation, 104, 107, 110, 112, 186–189
chemotherapy agents, 241
chest at breast position, 21
chest-to-chest position, 21
chicken pox, in mother, 167
children. *See* infants
cigarettes, 85, 94, 161–163, 218

classic galactosemia, 150–151
clavicle, broken, 155–156
cleft palate, 108, 147–150, 196
clutch posture, 192, 192*f*
colic and feeding issues, 137–139
collaborative breastfeeding,
   13–14, 14*f*, 16, 20
colostrum, 82, 128, 169
complementary feeding, 4–5
congenital breast anomalies, 85
Convention on the Rights
   of the Child, 253
conversion table, 277
convulsions, 142, 150
   for lactation, 7–11
counseling, for lactation. *See*
   lactation counseling
cow's milk, reaction to, 87, 151
cradle position, 100, 100*f*,
   190, 190*f*
craniofacial anomaly, and
   feeding issues, 148–149
cribs, 94
cross-cradle posture, 191, 191*f*
crying, 13, 77–78, 134–135, 142
   at breast, 112–115
   as feeding cues, 19
cup feeding, 3, 234
cynanosis, 142
cyst, in breast, 85. *See also*
   plugged duct

D

dairy, reaction to, 138
dehydration, of baby, 95, 98, 139
delivery staff, responsibilities
   of, 31–32
Department of Health and
   Human Services (HHS),
   243–244
Depo-Provera, 175
depression, 85
   postnatal, 245–248
diabetes, in mother, 141
diet, affecting breastmilk,
   86–87, 138
donor milk, 3, 59, 81
Down syndrome, and feeding
   issues, 145–147, 195–196
"down-under" posture, 58–59,
   59*f*, 89, 193, 194*f*, 224, 224*f*
drug use, and feeding, 85, 94,
   163–166, 241
"dry up" breast, 74

duarte galactosemia, 150–151
ducts
   plugged, 59, 66, 69–71, 75
   severed, 45

E

EBMF. *See* exclusive breastmilk
   feeding
eczema, 62, 87, 152
Edinburgh Postnatal Depression
   Scale (EPDS), 245–248
eggs, reaction to, 87
engorgement, 172–173
   breast and nipple issues
      resulting from, 43, 45–46,
      48–49, 74
   insufficient milk supply caused
      by, 84
   symptoms and solutions for,
      66–69, 67*f*
EPDS. *See* Edinburgh Postnatal
   Depression Scale
Epstein-Barr, 167
estrogen birth control, 175
everted nipple, 46, 47*f*
exclusive breastmilk feeding
   (EBMF), 1–3, 33, 86
eyes, opacity in, 150

F

facility staff, responsibilities
   of, 29–30
failure to thrive, 51
Fair Labor Standards Act, 91
family planning, 174–177
   natural. *See* symptothermal
   method
fat stores, maternal, 86
FDA. *See* Food and Drug
   Administration
fear, associated with
   breastfeeding, 40
feeding. *See also* feeding issues
   alternate methods of,
      129–131
   block, 89
   blue lips during, 110
   cues, 159
      identifying, 13, 35, 78–80,
         78–80*f*
      at night, 93
   for normal breastfeeding,
      17–20, 18–20*f*, 26*f*
   devices for, 3, 234, 285

duration of individual, 25, 120–121
first, 31
frequency of, 77–88
gassy after, 223
observation checklist, 104, 107, 110, 112, 186–189
"on demand," 77
problems with. *See* feeding issues; breastfeeding, management issues and
scheduled/delayed, 40, 98–99
spitting up after, 58, 151–152, 223
successful sequence of, 16–26
when to stop, 25, 25f, 171–174
feeding issues, 95–159. *See also* premature babies
birth injuries, 153–156
bottle/cup refusal, 129–131
cardiac birth defect, 108, 143–144
cessation of breastfeeding, early, 5
colic and, 87, 137–139
craniofacial anomaly, 148–149
crying at breast, 112–115, 134–135
detaching from breast, 106–108
Down syndrome, 145–147, 195–196
empty feeling breasts, 123–126
expressed milk, small quantity of, 126–129
falling sleeping at breast, 115
fretful baby, after feeding, 121–123
fretting, at breast, 109–111
galactosemia, 2, 150–151, 241
horses, zebras, or unicorns level of, 8–11
hypoglycemia, 120, 141–143
jaundice, 139–141, 150, 154
phenylketonuria, 2, 152–153
refusing to feed, 95–99
from one breast, 99–103
sleeping at breast, 13, 118–121
sleeping through night, 92–93, 132–134
sporadic refusing to feed, 103–106
waking up enough to nurse, 135–137
weight gain issues, 115–118

fever, 10, 66
first feeding, 31
fish, reaction to, 87
flaking skin, on nipple, 62–64
flange, of breast pump, 83–84
flat nipple, 46–48, 47f
flexing of arms and legs, as feeding cue, 17, 78, 79f
flu, 168
flu-like symptoms. *See* mastitis
fluconazole, 63
fontanelles, sunken, 139
Food and Drug Administration (FDA), 232
food reactions, 86–87, 138
football posture, 100, 100f, 192, 192f
formula
4-D pathway, 28
as addition to diet of baby, 4, 82
educating on use of, 33
marketing of, 33, 37–38, 40, 249–250
special, 2, 151
supplementing with, 169
weaning, use after, 172
frenulum stretches, 57
fretting, at breast, 109–111

G

gag reflex, of baby, 108, 223
galactocele, 74–75
galactosemia, 2
and feeding issues, 150–151, 241
gape, failure to, 22, 23f
garlic, 86
gassy foods, avoiding, 86
gastrointestinal problems, 138
Global Strategy for Infant and Young Child Feeding, 251–252
glossary of terms, 258–276
Goals for the United States, 243–244
growth curves/charts, 81, 84, 87–88, 116
guided imagery, expressing milk, 83
Guidelines: Breastfeeding, Family Planning, and the Lactational Amenorrhea Method—LAM (Labbok, Cooney, & Coly), 176f

H

hand expression, 127,
   230–231, 231*f*
hand-to-mouth, as feeding cue,
   19, 20*f*, 79, 80*f*
head birth injury, and feeding
   issues, 153–155
head plexus injury, 101, 113
Health Care Reform Bill
   (U.S.), 91
Health Education Associates, 88
Health Resources and Services
   Administration Office on
   Women's Health, 92
healthcare employees,
   responsibilities of
administrative staff, 37–38
facility staff, 29–30
labor and delivery staff, 31–32
maternity staff, 38
postpartum staff, 32–37
prenatal/antenatal staff, 30, 39
Healthy Children Project,
   Inc., 7. *See also* Center for
   Breastfeeding
Healthy People, U.S. objectives,
   1, 243–244
hemorrhage, postpartum, 218
hepatitis, mothers with, 167
herbal supplements, 164
herpes viruses, mothers
   with, 167
HHS. *See* Department
   of Health and Human
   Services
HIV positive mothers, 166,
   235–236, 241
HMBANA. *See* Human Milk
   Banking Association of
   North America
hormones
birth control, 175
problems, 85, 125, 218
hospitals and birth centers,
   27–38
artificial teat or pacifier, use
   of, 35–36
breastfeeding on demand,
   encouraging, 35–36
informing women of benefits
   of breastfeeding, 30
initiating breastfeeding after
   birth, 31–32

International Code of
   Marketing of Breast-Milk
   Substitutes compliance, 37
newborn, foods for, 33
rooming-in, practice of, 34
support groups, establishing,
   36–37
teaching breastfeeding, 32–33
training for policy
   implementation, 29–30
written policy for
   breastfeeding, 28–29
Human Milk Banking
   Association of North
   America (HMBANA), 3, 81
human rights, 253
human T-cell lymphotropic
   virus, 241
hunger, of infant, 13, 82, 98,
   115. *See also* feeding, cues
hyperactivity, in baby, 152
hyperthyroidism, 85
hypoglycemia, and feeding
   issues, 120, 141–143
hypothyroidism, 85, 219
hypotonia, 142

I

illness, breastfeeding during, 3,
   166–168
implants, breast, 43–45
individual care plans, for
   mother and baby, 37
Infant Risk Center, 164
infants
beds for, 94
contact needs of, 86, 120
daily milk needs of, 199–200, 220
discomfort at breast, 109–111
elimination patterns of, 88,
   217, 224
falling asleep, at breast, 13,
   118–121
forcing to feed, 97
hunger of, 13, 82, 98, 115
inadequate suck of, 40
mistakenly fed another's
   breastmilk, 235–236
newborns, 15–16, 33, 77–78,
   92–94
position at breast, 55, 62, 64.
   See also latch
safety, 93–94

sucking of. *See* sucking, of infant
warning signs, 287
weight
  checks, 44, 51
  expectations for, 80–81, 87,
    93, 217
  inadequate, 115–118
  loss, 81
  rapid gain, 58, 87–90, 223
  table for calculating loss,
    209–216
infection
  bacterial, 63–64
  of nipple, 62
infectious disease, of mother, 166
inflammation, in breast. *See*
  mastitis
influenza, 168
inhaler, 162
injury
  of baby during birth, 153–156.
    See also specific injuries
  to breast, 85, 218
Innocenti Declaration on Infant
  and Young Child Feeding
  (2005), 253–257
Institute of Medicine, 87
insufficient milk syndrome, 82
insulin, and milk supply, 85
International Code of
  Marketing of Breast-milk
  Substitutes, 37, 249–250
inverted nipple, 40, 49–52, 49*f*,
  218–219

J

jaundice, and feeding issues,
  139–141, 150, 154
jaw motion, and nutritive
  sucking, 188, 188*f*
Joint Commission, The, 3

L

labor and delivery staff,
  responsibilities of, 31–32
labor medications, 46
lactation counseling
  approach to, 7–11
  eight-level process, 181–185, 182*f*
lactation insufficiency. *See* milk
  supply adequacy
lactational amenorrhea (LAM),
  175, 176*f*

LactMed, database of drugs, 164
laid-back posture, 193, 193*f*
LAM. *See* lactational amenorrhea
latch, 14, 52–57, 56*f*, 63, 187, 187*f*
  asymmetric, 23, 24*f*, 48, 50
latch-off, shape of nipple after,
  14, 48, 51, 55–57, 223
late preterm infant (LPTI), 159
Lee, Nikki, 82
let-down, 128
  forceful, 193
lethargic baby, 140, 142, 150
lip color, during feeding, 110,
  147–148
LPTI. *See* late preterm infant
lumps, in breast, 69–71, 73
lyme disease, 167
lymph drainage, 69

M

Madonna posture, 190, 190*f*
malnutrition
  of baby, 4, 52, 77, 82–83, 95
  of mother, 85
marketing, of formula, 33, 37–38,
  40, 249–250
massage, 56, 96, 96*f*, 195–196, 195*f*
mastitis
  abscess caused by, 75
  breastfeeding and, 167
  mistaken for other conditions,
    10, 65–67, 70
  oversupply and, 88–89
  preventing, 59, 72–73, 172–173
  symptoms and solutions, 71–73
maternity staff, responsibilities
  of, 38
medication
  for abscess, 74
  breastfeeding while taking,
    3, 85, 163–166, 218
  co-sleeping and, 94
  feeding refusal and, 95, 105
  from labor, 15, 46
  for mastitis, 72
  safety resources, 285–286
  for yeast or thrush, 63
Medications and Mother's Milk
  (Hale), 164
menstrual period, and baby's
  refusal to feed, 105
methycillin-resistant *Staphylococcus
  aureus* (MRSA), 74

microcephaly, 152
milk bank, 3, 59, 81, 89
milk blister. *See* bleb
milk insufficiency
  actual, 83
  maternal reasons for, 84–85
  perceived, 82–83
milk supply adequacy
  assessing, 52, 226–229
  breast surgery affecting, 43–45
  empty feeling breasts and,
    123–126
  flow rate, 58, 218–222
  fretful baby after feeding and,
    121–123
  insufficient, 82–84
  inverted nipples and, 50
  poor weight gain and, 81,
    115–118
  sleeping at breast and, 118–121
  small quantity of expressed
    milk and, 126–129
milk supply building/relactation,
  protocol for, 218–222
milk transfer. *See* breastmilk,
  transfer
millennium development
  goals, 2
minerals, adding to baby's
  diet, 2–3
mood disorders, 85, 245–248
Moro reflex, 142
mother-led weaning, 171
mother–baby comfort
  assessment, 32
mother's diet, affecting
  breastmilk, 86–87
mouthing, as feeding cue, 17,
  19*f*, 79, 79*f*
MRSA. *See* methycillin-resistant
  Staphylococcus aureus
multiple babies, 177–179
muscle tone, in baby, 145, 146*f*

N

napping, 93
National Center for Health
  Statistics, 81, 87–88
National Library of Medicine
  (U.S.), 164
natural family planning. *See*
  symptothermal method

NCHS. *See* National Center for
  Health Statistics
neck birth injury, and feeding
  issues, 155–156
neuromuscular problems, 97, 108
newborn infants. *See* infants,
  newborns
nicotine patch, 162
nifedipine, 61
nipple, positions of, 22–24, 22–24*f*
nipple issues. *See* breast and
  nipple issues
nonnutritive sucking, 188, 188*f*
normal breastfeeding, 13–14
  getting started, 13–14
  positions for, 20–24, 21–24*f*
  self-attached, 15–16
  sequence of successful feeding,
    16–26
nursing strikes, 173
nutritional supplements, of
  mother, 164
nutritive sucking, 188, 188*f*
nystatin, 63

O

observation checklist, feeding,
  104, 107, 110, 112, 186–189
odor, of baby, 152
"on demand" feeding, 77
oral suspension, 63
over-the-counter medication,
  during breastfeeding,
  163–166
oxytocin, 111, 127

P

pacifiers, 35–36, 104, 218
Paget's disease, 73
pain
  while actively feeding, 14,
    52–57, 223
  after breastfeeding, 60–62
  constant burning, 62–64
  from oversupply, 57–60
  plugged duct or caked breast,
    69–71
  radiating through breast, 64–66
palate shape, in baby's mouth,
  57, 108, 147–150, 196
PCOS. *See* polycystic ovarian
  syndrome

perceived milk insufficiency, 82–83
phenylketonuria (PKU), 2
feeding issues, 152–153
Pierre Robin sequence, 147–150
pituitary infarct, 85
PKU. *See* phenylketonuria
placental fragments, retained, 85, 125, 128, 218
plexus injury, head or brachial, 101, 113, 155–156
plugged duct, 59, 66, 69–71, 75
pneumonia, aspiration, 155
policy on breastfeeding, of hospitals and birth centers, 28–29
polycystic ovarian syndrome (PCOS), 85, 125
postnatal depression, 245–248
postpartum hemorrhage, 218
postpartum staff, responsibilities of, 32–37
postpartum support, for breastfeeding, 36–37, 40–41
power pumping, 84
pregnancy
breastfeeding during, 169–171
hormones of, 170
and milk production, 85
prevention by breastfeeding, 174–177
premature babies
contraindications to exclusive breastfeeding, 2
expression of breastmilk for, 32–33
feeding issues and, 64, 156–159, 196
multiples, breastfeeding, 177
pacifiers, use of, 35–36
posture for feeding, 191, 229*f*
prenatal education, for mother, 30
prenatal staff, responsibilities of, 30, 39
prescription medications, 163–166
preterm babies. *See* premature babies
proctocolitis, 87
progestin-only birth control, 175

prolactin levels, in milk, 50
pseudoephedrine, 218

R

radiation treatment, and breastfeeding, 3, 163–164, 242
rapid eye movement (REM), 13, 17, 19*f*, 78, 79*f*
Raynaud's phenomenon, 60–62
reddened area, of breast. *See* mastitis
refusing bottle/cup, 129–131
relactation/building milk supply, protocol for, 218–222
REM. *See* rapid eye movement
respiratory problems, 97, 108, 110, 142
rooming-in, practice of, 34
rooting, as feeding cues, 17, 78, 78*f*
rule of 3 (colic), 137

S

searching movements, as feeding cues, 17, 78, 78*f*
secondhand smoke, 161–163
seizure, in baby, 142, 152
self-attached breastfeeding, 13, 14*f*, 15–16
semi-reclining posture, 193, 193*f*
sharing bed, with baby, 94
Sheehan's syndrome, 85
shell, breast, 51, 72
shiny skin, on nipple, 62–64
side-car sleepers, 94
side-lying posture, 193, 194*f*
SIDS. *See* sudden infant death syndrome
skin cancer, 3
skin color, during feeding, 110, 147–148
skin-to-skin holding
after birth, 31, 34
feeding problems, resolving, 97, 104, 107, 110
management issues and, 80
during normal breastfeeding, 15, 15*f*
sleep cycles, 80. *See also* rapid eye movement

sleeping
  at breast, 13, 115, 118–121
  close to mother, 93–94
  through night, 92–93, 132–134
sleepy baby, 51, 135–137, 142
smoking, 85, 94, 161–163, 218
society-led weaning, 171
solid foods, introduction of, 81,
    88, 154, 156
sore nipples, 169
soy, reaction to, 87
spicy foods, avoiding, 86
"spoiling" baby, 99
spoon feeding, 234
staff, healthcare. *See*
    healthcare employees,
    responsibilities of
"starving baby out," 131
strikes, nursing, 173
stunted growth, of baby, 4
subtle body motions, as feeding
    cues, 17, 18*f*
sucking, of infant
  inadequate, 196
  nonnutritive, 188, 188*f*
  sucking pattern, 23, 25
sudden infant death syndrome
    (SIDS), 94
sunlight exposure, and
    vitamin D, 3
surgery, breast. *See* breast surgery
swaddling, 14
swollen breasts. *See*
    engorgement
symptothermal method, 176
syringe feeding, 3

T

T-cell lymphotropic virus, 241
tandem nursing, 170
"tank up," 93
teething, 93, 113, 123, 133
temperature, of nipple, 61
theca lutein cyst, 85
thrive, failure to, 51
thrush, 61–64
thyroid/hormone problems,
    125, 218
tobacco use, 85, 94, 161–163, 218
tongue tie, 57, 72, 108
torticollis, 101
toxoplasmosis, 167
tremors, in baby, 152

triplets, ability to breastfeed,
    177–179
tuberculosis, 166, 241
tummy-to-tummy position, 21
twins, ability to breastfeed,
    177–179

U

unique identifiers, 9
UNICEF. *See* United Nations
    Children's Fund
United Nations Children's Fund
    (UNICEF)
  Baby-Friendly Hospital
    Initiative, 27
  Global Strategy for Infant
    and Young Child Feeding,
    251–252
  Innocenti Declaration on
    Infant and Young Children,
    253–257
  International Code of
    Marketing of Breast-milk
    Substitutes, 249
  on malnutrition, 4
  on sleep safety, 94
United States, goals for, 243–244

V

varicella-zoster, 167
vasospasm, of nipple, 60–62
vectors, treating for yeast, 63
venereal warts, 167
vitamins
  adding to baby's diet, 2–3
  taken by mother, 164
  vitamin D, 3
vomiting, after feeding, 58, 150,
    152, 223

W

water baths, for breast, 67, 68*f*
weaning, 170–174
websites, for support
    organizations, 278–286
weight gain/loss of baby. *See*
    infants, weight
weight loss table. *See* baby weight
    loss table
well-being, of mother, 86
wheat, reaction to, 87
white patches, in baby's mouth,
    62–64

WHO. *See* World Health
    Organization
World Health Assembly, 37, 249
World Health Organization
    (WHO)
  Baby-Friendly Hospital
    Initiative, 27
  Global Strategy for Infant
    and Young Child Feeding,
    251–252

growth curves, 81, 88
Innocenti Declaration on
    Infant and Young Children,
    253–257
recommendations of, 4
written policy, on breastfeeding,
    28–29

Y

yeast, 61–64